AWAKE AGAIN

AWAKE AGAIN

MARTIN KRIEG

WRS
PUBLISHING

A Division of WRS Group, Inc.
Waco, Texas

First published in the United States of America in 1994 by WRS Publishing, A Division of WRS Group, Inc., 701 N. New Road, Waco, Texas 76710
Book design by Kenneth Turbeville
Jacket design by Joe James

10 9 8 7 6 5 4 3 2 1

Library of Congress Cataloging-in-Publication Data

Krieg, Martin.
      Awake again/Martin Krieg.
           P.   cm.
      ISBN 1-56796-046-4 : $18.95
      1. Krieg, Martin—Health. 2. Brain damage—Patients—United States—Biography. I. Title.
RC387.5.K74 1994
362.1'97481—dc20
[B]

                                 94-3841
                                 CIP

Dedication

*To Andrea Susan Reich, CPA,
whose friendship and expertise
have authenticated the
National Bicycle Greenway.*

*10% of the royalties from each sale
of this book will be divided equally between
the National Bicycle Greenway and
the National Head Injury Foundation*

Table of Contents

Acknowledgments

THE LONG JOURNEY OF THANKS

To Jim Donovan, for his gracious direction, dedication to excellence, and for knowing exactly what my book needed.

To Don Chu, Ph.D., for helping me to find what I had inside of me.

To Uncles Dan and Jim Sanchez for introducing me to a different way of living.

To Karen Bauder for loving me so genuinely.

To Ron Swenson for helping me place my dreams before the business community.

To Andrea Hammett, who worked tirelessly to help me build a strong foundation.

To Jerry Annis, who helped me produce my first bicycle directories.

To Neil Wilkinson, who helped me get them printed.

To Bev Gordon, Dan Floyd, Dennis Nelson, Michelle Cavaleri, Georgia Schroer, Teresa Fitzpatrick, all, for investing in my books.

To Lee Dusic, who broadcast my dream.

To Dick Ryan for the example of his perseverance in building recumbent bicycles.

To Carin Hanna for so unselfishly supporting my work.

To Mark Gold, Esq., for always believing in the Greenway.

To Charlotte Riley, who laughed when it was hard.

To John A. Brown, whose successes remind me to keep my eye on the prize.

To Spiros Bairaktaris, who gave so many of his hours and talent in the very beginning.

To Sandy Mason, Gardner Martin, Jeanne Taylor, D.C., Dave Love, D.C., Karl Abbey, Michele Wilson, Carol Holdaway, Mark and Sandy Kemmerling, Terry and Connie Shaw, Dick Powell, Dan Bellick, and Tony Plotkin for keeping the Greenway dream alive.

To Jim Hatfield for being there to solve my computer mysteries.

To John Ryan for all the long hours that resulted in beautiful maps.

To Richard Curtis and Bob Page for helping me understand word authority.

To George Zitnay, Ph.D., for recognizing my ability to help the cause of head injury.

To Lisa and MaryRose Dzyban for bringing their genius to my book project.

To Colin Ingram for adding so much to my life, my writing, and to the Greenway project.

To Betsy Lyon for her example of polish, class, and warmth.

To Justine Gerbrandt for the gift of her beauty and for pushing me to a whole new level.

To Dave Giggy, whose courage and love I admire.

And to all those who believe in me, including Cyrus Oster, Tom, Susan and Edith Sullivan, Linda Mitchell, Gaylord Hill, Bob Pussey, Ron Goldin, Jerri Parrilla, Ross Shafer, Patti Craves, Alan and Hanz Scholz, the people of Santa Cruz, Angela Cadile, Dave and Sandy Geist, Mary Daffield, Greg Davis, Kent Garliep, John, Elza and Teresa at the SBDC, Jordan Bonfield, Julie Pelletier, Kieran Bahn, Marge and Bob Laxson, Gary Patton, Carla Price, Chris Angelini, Dale Wickenheiser, Dave Murawski, Birgette Karlson, Chris Vantornhout, Elaine Hebert, Jack Hildreth, Dierdre Smith, Dick and Jayne Murdock, Sara Gist, Matt Koue, Marvin and Bert Smith, Sandy Lesnewski, Darius and Denise Mohsenin, Rod Nagy, Lauren Basile, C.W. Swenson and Richard Cogura.

To the people at WRS Publishing, including Dr. Wayman Spence, Jary Ganske, Sherry Claypool, Kenneth Turbeville, Joe James, Ann Page, Mark Patz, Eileen Kenney, Reneé Selman, Judy Garrett and Brenda Roberts for being so full of love, and especially to Georgia Brady for her impeccable integrity and for her sensitivity to the book's needs.

To all the people in my past and present, and lastly…

To the Kriegs (all of you). Thanks for being a part of this grand journey with me. I love you all.

Foreword

The day of the accident, Martin Krieg lost his ability to think—to know who or what he or his family was, to know that he'd been hurt, or even to know that he had an identity separate from a hospital environment. From somewhere deep within, however, a voice asked if he wanted to live—and live a life that would inspire others. He responded to that question by "coming back" and showing us what any of us can do to improve our own lives.

As you read these pages, you will see how Martin learned the significance of James Allen's words—"Circumstances do not make the man, they reveal him"—as he traces through the events that lead up to, and follow, his car wreck. Suddenly forced to overcome tremendous mental and physical obstacles, he begins to understand how his every action fits into the bigger picture of his life. For example, the book you are reading now began fifteen years ago as Martin wrote to formulate his thoughts and feelings—to record and understand what had happened to him and the ways in which he was changed. Wanting to make the most of his new lease on life, he learned how to read again by reading and rereading the words of wise men and women, acknowledging the mysterious "connectedness" of us all and our influence on each other.

From his odyssey, you will begin to understand how thought affects the body. Martin tells how he learned to walk again by focusing his thought like a laser beam on the desired result. Always embracing the next challenge, he set goals for himself. He would not be satisfied until he overcame each and every one of his limitations and became a better person than he'd ever been.

It seems that Martin will never be completely satisfied that his rehabilitation is complete, and for that we can all be thankful. His desire to prove that his life was worth saving has resulted in his work toward the creation of The National Bicycle Greenway, which is now well underway. If this book is any indication of the strength of his determination, I feel that soon enough, many people across this nation will rally to his crusade. Martin's long journey back, of which I feel privileged to have been a part, proves that there really are no limits to what we can achieve with the right attitude.

—Wayne Dyer, Ph.D.
Author *Your Erroneous Zones, Real Magic*

Introduction

It has been my privilege to have been one of Martin Krieg's teachers on his road to wholeness. In *Awake Again*, Martin Krieg gives life to the words that motivational speakers and authors have used for years. In his book, he shows how any of us, when faced with what may seem to be insurmountable odds, can arise triumphant with the right mental tools.

Faced with a bleak prognosis for wellness, Martin got out there, made mistakes, went back to the drawing board of his books and tapes and learned and grew. He kept going until he started to get a few things right. His confidence started to build. Redefining himself as an injured athlete, instead of the sickly cripple he was, Martin started to have success. And he kept building on his successes until he reached his goal of being able to help those who had helped him.

Throughout the grand adventure that this book details, the reader will no doubt take inspiration from the success principles that Martin Krieg has made so much a part of his life. After you're done with this book, if you're like me, you'll begin to understand how real Martin's dream for the coast-to-coast bicycle highway he calls the National Bicycle Greenway really is.

My work as a motivational speaker feels so rewarding when I can read a book like *Awake Again*. Watching what one man has done to rebuild himself and what he continues to do for mankind, makes me feel honored to have been any part of it. I know the experience will truly inspire you as well.

—Denis Waitley, Ph.D.
Author, *Psychology Winning*

Chapter 1

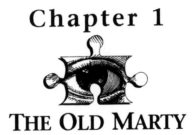

THE OLD MARTY

The bell signaling the end of P.E. rang. While others walked off the soccer field, I sprinted for the locker room. If I hurried, maybe I could get a shower before anyone saw me.

"Look at Krieg, he's hurrying so we won't see his little baby wienie," yelled Church.

Damn, I thought to myself. Busted. Very carefully, I slowed down.

By the time I got to be a senior, the rule, "All boys must take a shower after P.E.," was obnoxiously enforced by my peers. If I wrapped a towel around myself as I walked to or from the showers, a wisecracker would always point out that I was hiding my lack of body hair.

I tried different strategies. For a few weeks, I just got my hair wet with my comb and splashed water on my face to make it look like I had complied with the appropriate code of conduct. But when Mastro complained to one of the coaches about my scheme, everyone began to keep a close eye on me whenever I was near a sink. I tried walking to the shower stalls with my street pants on. If I stayed very close to the overlooking window of the coaches' office, no one inside could see that I was still partly dressed. Once I made it to the showers, I stalled. I acted like I had left something behind, then headed back to my locker. Sometimes it worked, sometimes it didn't.

I couldn't seem to escape the persecution caused by my classmates' fascination with hair—or the lack of it. I was only five feet, two inches and weighed a slight 108 pounds. I was insecure enough as it was. Having the body hair of a newborn baby didn't help my confidence one bit.

I began to lie awake wondering when God would grant me passage into manhood. I was eighteen years old and a senior, after all. It was 1971 and I would graduate from Moreau High School, an all-boys Catholic school in my hometown of Hayward, California, that spring. I wanted to grow tall, acquire a deep voice, and have lots of body hair. Running out of ways to disguise my physical immaturity, I refined the science of proper towel-holding. I developed a strict set of rules—Krieg's Humiliation-Avoidance Techniques. One, always dress or undress facing your locker. Two, don't, for any reason, turn sideways. Three, don't be caught off guard by anyone trying to get your attention. Four, use a shower nozzle against a corner. (If a nozzle that satisfies this criteria is not available, stall until one is.) Five, walk (don't run) to or from the showers, always keeping a wall about a foot away. This method keeps advancing onlookers from overtaking you on the exposed side. Six, on your exposed side, drape your towel over your clutched hand and hold it near your hip, six to eight inches in front of your body as you walk. Try to play cool—don't make it look like you're holding a bullfighter's cape. And seven, if a head-on encounter threatens, quickly shift both your towel and body to the appropriate side.

To lower my odds of being seen, I always waited until the last moment to take a shower. I watched the clock. I rearranged my locker. I tied my shoes. I combed my hair. Very slowly. All the while, I kept my peers distracted from the fact that I was not undressing by following another set of rules—Krieg's Keep-Them-Off-Guard Stall. One, crack jokes about Father Near's history class. Two, loudly debate which team would have won if the bell hadn't ended class. Three, tell stories about your wild bicycle camping trips. And four, make opinionated comments about the Oakland Raiders' latest draft selections.

Then, when almost everyone had filtered out of the smelly locker room, I would express alarm that I hadn't taken a shower yet. Quickly disrobing, I would make a quick dash to the showers, carefully holding my towel the correct way both coming and going.

Somehow I sensed that my persecution was preparing me for far greater challenges. I did not, however, make it any easier on myself by being the only bicycle commuter at my high school.

"And what are these things?" Keyes, an underclassman, asked the next morning in front of the school cafeteria. We all went by last names at Moreau.

"They're quick-release levers for taking off the wheels."

"What, you just pull on 'em and the wheel comes off?" Keyes looked away to the steady procession of cars that rumbled through the alleyway. As doors opened and closed, and engines stopped and started, kids carrying textbooks scampered in a hundred different directions.

"Yeah. Pretty cool, huh?"

"Not bad, Krieg." Keyes was impressed.

"Hi, Marty," John Hartin's mom called out as she stopped to let off her twin boys, John and Jim, for school. "Did you get a new bike?"

"Sure did, Mrs. Hartin," I said, "I'm showing it to Jeff right now."

"Gonna use it on your paper route?" John asked as he and Jim quickly joined the other students hanging around in front of the cafeteria. I nodded.

Small, freckle-faced redheads, the twins stayed as far away from my bike as possible. Even though they were my friends, they did not want to face any unneeded embarrassment by being associated with me when my bike was around. I usually locked it to a tree in the backyard of the church rectory, just across the parking lot from the breezeway where a lot of kids collected before school.

"Well, you be careful," Mrs. Hartin said as she pulled out of the driveway to let other cars through.

"Look at little Krieg, he's showing off his new car," called Schindler from across the driveway where John and Jim now stood. He was a large loudmouth, one of the worst.

"Did little Marty get a new bicycle?" another voice teased.

The small group that had assembled to taunt me broke out in laughter. Keyes slid into the background.

They towered over me on the sidewalk. I stood all alone. Their deep, manly voices intimidated me.

"At least it's good for the environment," I said in my little boy's voice.

"At least it's good for the environment," Schindler mocked. "What's that? Krieg, you're weird. Why don't you go read in the library like you always do?" More laughter.

"Krieg, why don't you admit that you're just too short to see over a car dashboard," Avo chimed in. His real name was too long, so it had been shortened to Avo. The laughter increased.

"No, I'm not, I can... "

"You know what he's got that rack on the back for?"

Silva interrupted. "He's gonna pack his date for the senior ball on it."

"No, that's only if he finds a girl shorter than him," Morris cracked. The rest of the crowd was in hysterics at these witticisms.

I couldn't remember a day more humiliating—and school hadn't even started. I wanted to cry.

Did it really require a car to be accepted, I wondered? Would that make up for my lack of pubic hair or size? Prior to high school, getting good grades had made me a big shot. That was before my peers began owning their four-wheeled status symbols.

But my financial priorities had not changed since junior high school. While my contemporaries were buying mag wheels and four-barrel carburetors, I was still purchasing baseball cards, comic books, and bicycle accessories.

But that would change.

By the time I got to be a junior at Cal State Hayward, I gave in to the pressure. I bought a motorcycle with my paper route money. And the hecklers in high school were right. Though I wasn't much taller, 5'6" by this time, girls suddenly began to respond to me, though I still had almost no body hair. There were some girls, however, who didn't like motorcycles, so I took a part-time job so that I could also buy a used sports car, a '66 Triumph Spitfire. I made sure to buy one that ran but needed work, so that my friends could see me working on my wheels.

Soon, however, I spent more time working on my car than I spent with my friends or the girls it was intended to attract.

"Hey, Marty," Bobby, the kid next door, called one morning. "Are those your legs under there?"

"What's up, Bobby?"

"I was wondering if you knew anything about Gitanes. I'm thinking about getting one."

"That's what that Interclub is that's hanging in the garage," I said as I slid out from under the car, making sure to collect as much grease as I could. We both looked over at the bicycle that I used to spend many hours on.

"Don't you ride it any more? All I ever see you doing is working on your car." Bobby always wore a white T-shirt. His large stomach always made it look too small for him.

Inside I smiled. I wanted to be seen doing a man's job. Little boys don't work on cars, men do.

"You really oughta be riding your bike," Bobby continued. "Everyone's getting into it. My dad's even thinking about getting a bike and we wanted to ask you what you thought."

The gas crises of the early seventies had hit. Bicycles had arrived. And here I was stuck trying to prove my manhood with a car.

"Man, I gotta get my car running right so I can get to work. I don't have time for bicycles anymore," I said.

How ironic, I thought. I only worked two jobs so that I could support my car and motorcycle.

"Wanna sell it?" Bobby asked.

"I still get out once in a while."

"I never see you on it."

"Well, yeah, once in a while I throw it in the back of my car and drive out to Pleasanton where there ain't no cars and I just do sprints out there on the farm roads."

"Why, you afraid of cars? We always used to see your head going in and out of traffic."

"I'm not afraid of cars, I've just been riding so long, I need a little variety, that's all." I didn't want to admit that I would rather be cycling. I just didn't want to be part of the latest fad. So here I was trapped under the symbol of my manhood's hood. "Tell you what. You wanna ride with me on my motorcycle down to Foreign Auto? I've got to pick up some parts they ordered for me."

"No way, Marty, you're too crazy. I saw you scaring the shit out of Danny's sister the other day."

"Aw, she just likes to scream."

"Can you blame her?"

"Whattaya mean?"

"You got her sitting on the back while you're standing on the seat going forty miles an hour."

"Twenty miles an hour."

"Whatever. You know if you crash at just five miles an hour, someone's gonna get hurt. Oh yeah—my mom says she's gonna call the police if she sees you riding a wheelie when Michael or any of the other little kids are out here playing, just so you know."

"Huh." Mission accomplished! People call the police on men that do dangerous things on motorcycles. And they call them crazy. Yet on a bicycle no one ever notices you, and if they do they just think you're a harmless little fairy.

As Bobby walked away, a shiny-new gold Camaro turned the corner and stopped at the edge of my driveway.

"Hey, Krieg," Bob Beaudry called from the window as he revved the motor. "Wanna go water-skiing tomorrow?"

Bob's identity was so tied in to his car that he got out of it only when absolutely necessary. Only his muscled arm, rolled-up T-shirted shoulder, and head, dominated by incredibly long sideburns, stuck out of the window. Bob was a stud.

"Any chicks going?" I tried not to sound too excited.

Once Bob had told me that girls didn't care about how much hair boys have on their legs. So, as long as I kept my underarms and genitals from view, I could go to the rivers and lakes with Bob; neither he nor the girls we brought along would have to know about my problem. Almost out of college and still almost hairless.

"You know I never have any luck. I thought I'd see if you could put that together. See if Joan and her sister want to go."

"Who, Ussery? I ain't gonna ask her, she gave me shit at Blackmare's party last night."

"Come on, you can find a couple of girls for us. I'll call you tonight," Bob said as he backed his car up.

"What if they say they can't camp up there with us?"

"Talk 'em into it. Come on, Krieg, you're good at that. I gotta go."

Somehow, in a few years' time, my reputation was changing from a bicycle nerd to a ladies' man. I liked that. And 324 Ambrose Court where I lived was getting to be known as the cool place to visit. My new friends knew that they could work on their cars in my driveway and that they could use my tools. And all it took was a car.

A short while after Bob left, a tremendous explosion of automotive horsepower erupted a few blocks away. Engine thunder shattered the silence of our quiet neighborhood cul-de-sac. Tires screamed against asphalt, and a cloud of smoke enveloped the rear end of the approaching car.

Finally the driver let off the gas. It was Jeff Limbeck, in his souped-up 1964 Ford Fairlane. The Hyper 289 engine calmed to a low roar. Jeff coasted the rest of the way to my grease-stained driveway. He was laughing as he stopped and climbed from his car.

"Hey, Krieg, how'd you like that? I think your neighbor there in that brown house was yelling at me."

I looked to where he was pointing, then shook my head.

"You're crazy, Limbeck."

Even standing still, Jeff's Fairlane looked fast—and dangerous. So that he could run wider tires, he'd cut out the fenders with a hacksaw. Instead of then making the job look clean by filling the damaged area with Bondo, he simply spray-painted the jagged edges with flat black paint. He cut a gaping hole in the hood where the carburetor rose out of it. The passenger compartment teetered high above the chassis, exposing headers, exhaust pipes, and show-quality chromed wheel covers, nuts, bolts, and springs.

Like Bob's, Jeff's car was an extension of both his personality and his looks. While black electrical tape held Jeff's glasses together, paint-stained cutoffs revealed tan, muscular legs. Jeff's powerful shoulders and arms dwarfed the faded black T-shirt he wore. Brown, tightly curled hair that was long and parted at the side added to his incongruous looks.

"So. Where's the parties at tonight, Krieg? Rothskie says he saw you at Grand Auto and you told him about two up on Hillcrest."

"Well, there's those two. Krantz came by and told me about one up on Center that sounds pretty good."

"What time we gonna meet here?"

"I don't know, we're probably gonna take off around nine or ten. And my brother will be here with his goofy friends." Chris was a year younger than me but several inches taller. It bothered me.

"Chris's friends aren't that goofy. Why don't we just party here?"

"There ain't gonna be any girls."

"Well, how 'bout your sisters? You got three of 'em. Hell, Krieg, you're so tight, you never let them come around so we can talk to them."

"Gimme a break, Lim. Karen's only nine, and besides, they're my sisters. What fun is that?"

"Hey, your little sister's gonna grow up some day, and I want to be on good terms with her just in case. But I'm talking about Kathy and Nancy. They're both foxes, in case you hadn't noticed. All the guys are talking about 'em."

I ignored him. "Come back at eight. And don't forget to

bring some beer." I paused. Jeff never had any money, and he was a year younger than me, which meant he would have to prove he was old enough to buy. "You've got ID, don't you?"

He grinned. "Krieg, you think I need ID? Just because they card you everywhere you go doesn't mean they're gonna card me. Especially if I don't go with you."

I understood. Embarrassed, I changed the subject. "Hey, let's do goobers tonight. Here's two bucks. Get the ones that are salted in the shell."

"Wanna see another power stand?"

"No way, Limskie. I gotta live here. Just come back at eight with some beer."

"Just cause your little Spitfire can't burn rubber."

"How long can you go on a tank of gas? You can just about make it to the gas station, right?"

"Who cares, you worried about thirty or forty cents a gallon?"

"Hey, I don't believe in spending my life in gas lines or polluting the air. Besides, I'll bet more chicks would rather ride in my car than in yours."

"Wimpy cars get wimpy chicks. I like power cars and power chicks," Jeff yelled as he drove away.

Jeff's harmless comment saw right through my attempts to prove my manhood. I secretly hoped that my future career as an accountant would not be exposed in the same way. Instead of taking a major that was fun, I studied about boring balance sheets and profit-and-loss statements, because those who manage money command a respect that transcends physical limitations. Even with all my insecurities I could see that.

I could not, however, escape the downward spiral of four years of weekend carousing and partying once I actually took the job for which college had trained me. Even after I had worked a year as an accountant, my friends kept the pressure on.

"You gonna come out with me and Lim tonight, Krieg, or are you too good for us now?" Bob said one summer afternoon in 1977. "Dale says he saw you driving down Jackson with a tie on." That reduced Bob to cackling.

He and Jeff had stopped by the house that my brother and I shared—incidentally, the house where we had grown up. My parents and sisters had moved out and we had moved back in.

I wanted to distance myself from my old life, but I didn't want to hurt my two best friends from college.

"I'll rock and roll with you guys, but if we're gonna go over to Sunset tomorrow to play basketball, I've got to get in before midnight. I gotta help set up for inventory for a few hours tomorrow morning."

"Inventory! You trying to be a big shot on us, Krieg?" Bob never stopped teasing, but his teasing just didn't have the power it once had. Though he hadn't graduated from college yet, he worked forty hours a week at the local airport and had a pilot's license. He flew regularly. He imagined himself as a pilot for a large airline and never stopped telling us how pilots did and didn't act.

"Gee, Bob, do you even know what inventory means?"

"Sure, wiseguy, but since when do you work on Saturday mornings?"

"It's just part of my job. I have to go in on weekends once in a while or weeknights if they need me. I'm on salary now."

"Just don't forget who your friends are, Krieg, and who got you into water-skiing. And who took you for airplane rides."

Jeff laughed. "I remember when I took Krieg to his first party. Man, he was so nervous."

"Yeah, Krieg, and how many times did Lim protect you from fights?" Bob volunteered.

"All right, already. I guess I can stay out later," I relented. I wondered if I would ever be able to abandon the dual life I had been leading for the last year. When would I relinquish my college buddies and their lives of parties, cars, and girls for a more mature existence? Part of me wanted to. But part of me couldn't—or wouldn't—resist that carefree existence.

A phone call later that evening would help me find out.

I was studying my boss's notes on the next day's inventory when the phone rang. It was Jeff.

"Did you hear what happened to Mark?" Jeff's voice sounded urgent. "His company car blew up on him, and he's hurt pretty bad. We're all gonna meet at Dale's house tomorrow and then go over to the hospital to see him."

Mark Ramirez and I were a lot alike. Both of us were small and wiry, and we both tried to offset our lack of size—

and what we translated that to mean, a lack of virility—by being the life of every party. We weren't close friends, but I liked him.

"What do you mean, blew up?"

"The gas tank exploded on him. He was driving his company car, the one that runs on propane, and the thing blew up on him at the gas station."

"So what happened to him?"

"His brother was saying that he got burned over eighty percent of his body. They gotta scrub him every few hours to keep it all clean. He's conscious and all, but I wouldn't want to take that pain. But he's been handling it pretty well."

"I can't make it tomorrow, I'm going out to dinner with a couple of my college buddies. Then Sunday I'm supposed to pick up that BMW I'm buying... What hospital is he in? I'll go see him Monday when I get off."

"He's in this special burn hospital in Berkeley called Alta Bates, but you gotta be a family member to get in. You look like him—just say you're his brother. That's what we're gonna do, something like that." He paused. "Krieg, don't forget to see him. He needs all the support he can get. He's a man."

I wondered what had changed Jeff's opinion about Mark. Before the accident he would get on Mark's case even worse than mine. I found out Monday.

I drove out to Berkeley after work. A nurse ushered me into the small room where Mark lay watching TV. His disfigured face and blackened arms were a shock, but his voice was cheerful.

"What a surprise." His puffy lips muffled the words.

"Man... from what I heard I thought you wouldn't be coherent, what with all the drugs," I blurted out.

"Aw, you know how people are. They like to make things sound worse than they are."

I couldn't believe my eyes. Fun-loving Mark was now encased in black, puss-filled flesh. It was almost too much to look at. But we talked for a while about his accident and how he was getting along. Then another nurse came in.

"Excuse us, sir, but we have to clean Mark's wounds," she said.

Mark smiled, or tried to. "More torture... Marty, say hello to everyone for me. Tell them I'll be out in a few weeks, okay?" He looked at the nurse as she helped him into a wheelchair, as if seeking corroboration.

"If he can keep his good attitude so we can keep his burns clean, he'll be out pretty soon," she said.

"Bye, Mark."

"See you soon, Marty."

As the weeks passed, reports kept circulating about Mark's successful rehabilitation. No observation failed to mention how tough the little guy was, how he was "taking it like a man." I was almost envious of Mark. He had been given an opportunity to show what he was made of, what a man he was. He had triumphed over his lack of height.

A few months later I got my own chance.

I arranged a trip down the "River of No Return," the famous Salmon River in Idaho, and persuaded my brother Chris to go with me. Neither of us had ever gone down a river before, but I had seen an ad in the local paper for an organized river-rafting group. It seemed both dangerous and controlled at the same time. It would be my first paid vacation as an accountant.

Dad sensed that something was up. He took us out to dinner the night before we left to find out about the logistics of our trip.

"Now what I want to know is, how many days are you boys planning to get up to Idaho?" Dad seemed more serious than he usually was.

Chris looked at me. "We'll be there Saturday morning. It's only a day away," he answered.

"A day away if you're driving like maniacs. It's at least thirteen or fourteen hours. Aren't you two going to stop and rest anywhere?"

"Aw, come on, Dad. We're tough. We're young, we don't need rest like you. We'll trade places if one of us gets tired," I said.

Dad shook his head. He held his fork up to his eyes with his thick, work-hardened hands. He'd been a plumber for more than twenty years. Looking at the fork, he said, "I'm only going to say this once. Be careful. I don't like you kids taking this trip so nonchalantly. I also don't know why if this river trip doesn't start till Monday you have to be up there Saturday."

Chris put on his most mature face. "I know what you're worried about, Dad. Marty's got this thing about the River of No Return that he's been telling everybody about. I just tell people we're going rafting on the Salmon River. It's no big deal. We'll be okay."

"Whose car are you taking up there?"

"Marty's too cheap to take his."

"Hey, I'm paying for gas, what's the big deal?" I shot back.

Dad looked at me. "What's the big deal? Marty, you've got this fancy BMW parked in the driveway and you're gonna make your brother, who doesn't make half of what you make, take his bucket of bolts up there?"

"It's not a bucket of bolts," Chris said.

"You certainly don't think your Mustang is going to make it all the way up to Idaho without breaking down, do you? It bothers me just to see you hot-rodding around town in it," Dad said.

"Come on, Dad. I just put new tires on it and this last week I changed all the belts and spark plug cables. It's ready."

"I still don't know what the hell is wrong with Marty's car."

I thought quickly. "I haven't had time to get it all checked out," I said. "Besides, me and Chris never go anywhere in his car." What I really wanted was adventure, and Chris's red '66 Ford Fastback was fast, fun, and unpredictable.

Dad said softly, "Well, maybe it's good that you don't. Chris likes to hot-rod and neither of you needs to be egging the other on. I know how you two can get when you're together. I wish you'd spend more time with Janice, Marty. She seems pretty nice."

Janice and I had been going out off and on for a couple of years. But she was now going to Chico State, a couple hours north, and living on campus. We didn't really spend much time together anymore, and in truth we were just about broken up. I changed the subject as quickly as I could.

We talked about other things, then we went home and got a good night's sleep. After all, we'd be on the road for at least fourteen hours.

We left the next morning, about eight. The date was August 20, 1977.

Fourteen hours later we were lost.

We'd made good time, but we'd been on the road all day, not counting food and gas and rest breaks. But a few hours back we'd decided to take a short cut that I'd seen on the map. Somehow we'd wandered onto an Indian reservation, and we'd been trying to get off it for a couple hours, driving down an unlit dirt road that never seemed to end. We knew we couldn't be far from Boise, though. Chris had been driving for a while. He'd been ragging on me for the better part of an hour. "We just had to take a shortcut, Mr. Cornball."

"Don't blame me," I said. I had temporarily given up trying to find us on the map. "You thought it was a good idea, too, at the time. I wasn't the only one that..."

"Yeah, but you're the navigator. It's your job to figure out where we are and what the best route is... Wait a second. What's that up ahead?"

"I don't know... looks like an intersection. Maybe it's a real road."

"It's about time."

We were approaching the new road at an angle. We were moving pretty fast and almost there. "C'mon, Chris, slow down—is that a stop sign?"

"Yeah, but it's not for us. Don't worry, it's clear."

We bounced onto the new road at full speed. Out of nowhere there were lights and a blaring horn and screaming tires. And that was it. After that, nothing.

Seven weeks later, I slowly began to awaken from a coma. I was a two-year-old again, and might be one for the rest of my life.

Chapter 2

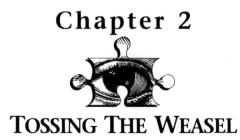

TOSSING THE WEASEL

It seemed like I had been asleep for a long, long time.

"Hello, Marty. I've heard a lot about you. My name is Sara and I'm going to help you learn how to talk again." For a long time there had just been one dull buzz in my head. For the first time a voice was distinct and understandable— and for the first time it seemed to matter to me. Her voice was bright and cheery as she wheeled me into her tiny office.

Sara's clear blue eyes put me into an immediate trance. I hadn't known that the moving shapes in my room were different from one another, that they weren't the same. Soft auburn curls framed her heart-shaped face. Her angelic voice spoke directly to my heart.

"You've got everyone quite worried because you haven't said anything for weeks, but I think there's someone inside," Sara said, and waited for me to agree.

I honestly did not know what she was talking about. Weeks? I didn't understand. I thought everyone understood me just fine, and I told her so with my eyes.

"Well, okay, Marty. If you really can talk, let me hear you say my name. I'm Sara, remember?"

I nodded as if I had completed the task.

"Have you said my name? I haven't heard anything yet."

What was she talking about? Couldn't she see what I had just communicated to her?

She seemed to sense my confusion. "Okay, Marty, how about if we do a little experiment? Will you do that with me?"

I wanted to impress her more than anything else in the world. Magic filled the air as her eyes sparkled with the excitement of the moment. I nodded.

"Great. Now I want you to breathe in as hard as you can. Let's try that a few times."

We inhaled together a few times. "Okay, now when you

exhale I want you to say 'seh'... " I inhaled, exhaled, and then said, "seh." "Let's try it again. You didn't say anything. I'll do it with you this time."

What was she talking about? I had just said "seh." I craved attention from this hypnotic woman, however, so I decided I would just play her game.

We inhaled together. "Now as you exhale go like this, seh... "

I looked at her, then exhaled, trying as hard as I could to say "seh." The sound that vibrated within my skull startled even me.

I looked at her as if I had done something wrong. A hazy memory told me that the last time I had experienced that sensation, a male nurse had slapped me for swearing at him.

"All right, Marty, I knew you had it in you." Sara's smile was wide. "Let's say the rest of my name, okay?"

She was my whole world, and I was eager to please her again. I nodded excitedly. "Okay, here's what you do. We're going to talk in syllables. My name is two sounds. It's 'Ser' and 'uh,' but you've got to put them together. Do you know how to do that?"

My eyes told her I did not.

"First let's breathe in, then 'Ser' as we exhale, and then without pausing, let's see you breathe in and breathe out 'uh.'"

I followed her instructions. It was hard work, but before long I was not only saying her name but had even said my own.

The excitement of the moment and all of the possibilities of actually speaking pounded inside my head and wore me out. I could not keep my eyes open. I slumped forward in my wheelchair, exhausted. It had been a long day.

Sara's voice softened. "Marty, that's going to be it for today. Tomorrow we'll show you how to talk in sentences. Let's get you back to your room."

As I lay half asleep in my bed, certain questions began to answer themselves. It seemed like the first time I'd been fully awake in an eternity. Maybe my inability to speak was why that woman who had come to see me had run out of the room with tears in her eyes when I thought we were communicating just fine. Shelly, my secretary at work who had visited me several times, had probably cried every time we'd "talked" for the same reason. It seemed to make sense now why no one paid attention to me when I said my feet were cold or that I had to go to the bathroom or that the water in the shower was too hot or too cold.

After a couple of days of learning how to work with my breath to join words together to form sentences, Sara said the words which would open up a whole new world for me. "Marty, I want you to talk at every opportunity you get. You haven't spoken for a really long time, so it's all going to take some practice. Will you do that for me?"

"Tawk... Okay?" I used my eyes to make a question out of my monotone words.

"That's right, Marty, don't be embarrassed. Don't get upset if people can't hear you either. It's just going to take time before you can project your voice. You punctured your lung, and it'll be a while before your lung capacity returns to normal, that's all. I want you to talk, talk, talk. Ask questions. Be curious. Learn about your world. Demand to know. The more you practice speaking again, the faster your words will get."

Sara had returned the world to me. She had given me back my name, which meant I was an individual whose feelings mattered. Also, because of her, I now possessed the keys to knowledge.

The first thing I wanted to know was why I was even in this place.

"Why... am... I... heh?" I asked. Sara watched eagerly as I forced each word out.

"You want to know why you're here in therapy?"

"Why," I begged.

"Marty, when your father comes to see you tonight, why don't you surprise him with that question. I'm sure he'd love to hear you talk," Sara said. I would find out later why she had avoided answering.

She really did want me to take my newfound ability to speak out of the safety of her office. That frightened me.

I slept the rest of the day. Dad, as always, arrived before anyone else. It was good to see his face. He sat down next to me.

"Boy, you wouldn't believe the job I worked today. I sure wish I had you. Remember those ditches you used to dig? I had to run one today, must've been twenty feet. Remember when you used to hit rock? You used to be one tough little guy, boy you'd get that pick going. I sure wish I had you today. And then they've got this damn plastic pipe they want us to run. Remember how I used to complain about them putting that stuff in? Well, this whole job is plastic pipe... " He continued a one-sided conversation about his workday as a plumber. "So how're things going today, podner?" Dad asked. I could tell he hadn't expected an answer. I hadn't said anything to him in weeks.

"Heeeyy... Da," I said. I watched as his eyes grew wide. He leaned closer to my bed.

"Son, you're talking! I don't believe it!" He trembled as he continued. "Did you want to say something, son?"

"Why... am... I... heh?" The stilted words came out in a hoarse whisper. Dad nodded as I said each word.

"Are you asking me why you're here?"

"Yeh... " I pleaded for him to continue with my eyes. My palms had broken into a sweat. The concentration required for speaking drained me. I fought to stay awake.

"Son, you don't know why you're here?" Dad was obviously disturbed. "You and your brother got into a very serious car wreck. Do you remember that river trip you boys were planning?"

My brother... a river trip... I vaguely remembered something of the sort. "Wha... " I forced out my surprise.

"Well, you kids never quite made it. Apparently Chris ran a stop sign and a trailer-truck ran right into your side of the car. Chris made it out with a few stitches and some pretty bad bruises... but do you even know you're in a hospital? Do you know your right side is paralyzed?"

"No... "

"Do you think that your wheelchair is normal stuff? What the heck do you think all these other people are doing in these beds?" Dad's face was twisted as he looked around my room. He was unable to comprehend my obvious frustration. He seemed angry that I could accept any of this. "You've got to be kidding me, Son—you don't even know where you're at? Let me see you move this arm if you think you're fine," he pointed to my right arm.

I nodded when I had completed the task.

"You think that's moving your arm? I didn't see it go anywhere. Make it do this," Dad said as he raised and lowered his hand.

Once again, I nodded.

"Son, you haven't moved anything. You're paralyzed." I was confused. I had thought that speaking would greatly please Dad. After all, back in Sara's safe little office, my every word had been praised.

So, just as I had done for Sara, I showed my father that I knew the names of the various objects in my room. After helping me say the words "newspaper," "flower," and "greeting card," Dad's voice shook as he said, "Son, I'm so glad to hear you can talk again. I just want you to know how much we're all rooting for you and how much you're loved. You're doing great. You're making great progress... I've got to go now." He grabbed my hand, then quickly got up to go. I could see the tears in his eyes before he turned away.

He left that evening both happy and sad, I think. I had proven to him that there was someone alive inside—but it was clear that, like a small child, I would have to start all over again.

As speaking slowly reorganized my mind, I began to dimly understand the discussions that went on among my many nightly visitors. I was fortunate just to be alive. I had been in four hospitals in six weeks. I had been in a general hospital in Boise, Idaho, for two weeks after the wreck, then been air-ambulanced to Eden Hospital in Castro Valley for two more weeks. I had spent two weeks at the University of California at San Francisco overlooking the Golden Gate Bridge; that's where I had finally started waking up. I was now in Fairmont Hospital, a rehab center.

I had been declared clinically dead back in Boise, and a priest had said last rites over me. Then, at Eden, I had almost lost my right leg when an arterial bleed in my thigh had gone undetected and had bled into the surrounding area. But my mother had fought against that; that's when I was moved to UCSF, one of the best hospitals in the nation, where teams of doctors monitored me around the clock for the two weeks I was there. UCSF was known for reversing hopeless cases, and they saved my leg.

But because of cerebral damage, my mental abilities had been impaired; the people here at Fairmont estimated my faculties to be those of a two-year-old child. My right side was paralyzed, and I had a punctured lung. The general prognosis was that I'd have to spend the rest of my life in a nursing home—if I survived.

It was overwhelming news, but it didn't really have much impact on me. In my mind's simple state, things seemed uncomplicated. All I knew was that another world seemed to exist on the outside of these white walls. And if that were so, maybe I could leave with people when they left. I resolved to ask Chris, my younger brother, how I could do that.

He showed up the next morning. It was the first time he'd visited me while I was fully conscious—semiconscious, anyway. It was the first time I could talk to him since the accident, and the first time he could talk to me. He looked at me, and his eyes filled with tears.

"Marty... I'm so sorry... "

What was he talking about? I was confused.

"Don't you remember that stop sign?"

I looked away. His anguish was so strong that it even pierced through the haze in my head.

"Do you remember anything? No? Well, I ran a stop sign. I thought it was for the other road. I went straight through it and that's when this four-ton trailer truck ran right into your side of the car. He was going fifty miles an hour. When everything stopped, I was all right." He paused. "But when I looked over at you, you weren't moving. I lost it."

He took a breath. "The guy in the truck had a CB, so he called for help. Caldwell wasn't too far away, and the paramedics got there pretty soon. They pulled you out through the rear window. That's when you suffered a heart seizure. They didn't think you were going to make it. The funny thing was, I thought you were all right at first. There wasn't much blood.

"I didn't think about the injuries being internal." He came closer and took my hand. "Can you forgive me?"

I still didn't know what he was talking about. There was only one thing I could remember in my woozy state.

"Hey... Kwiss... how... dooo... I... get... out... heh?" I could tell that my words lacked inflection. They were monotone. I used my eyes to help Chris feel the urgency of my request.

Chris's face was a study in concentration as he tried to assign meaning to the garbled words I was using. Finally he understood.

"What, you want to get out? You want to know how to get out?" he said excitedly.

"How... " I deadpanned.

"Marty... Man, you've got to really start doing your therapy the best you can."

"What... therr... pee?"

Chris's eyes moved away from mine.

"Marty, that's what those nurses are doing when they ask you to stack those little building blocks on top of each other. Your motor skills got knocked out, that's why you get food all over yourself when you try to eat. Haven't you ever noticed that you're pretty dangerous with a fork?" Chris laughed.

Without waiting for me to acknowledge him, he continued, this time more softly. "Marty, you've got all kinds of things to work on. You've really got to try when they ask you to push against their arms or throw bean bags. If you give it your best shot, pretty soon you'll be able to dress yourself and tie your own shoes. You don't want someone doing that for you the rest of your life, do you?"

I knew that people who came from the outside could walk. That's all I knew. I asked, "How... wok?"

"Well, you've got to really try hard from now on if you want to be able to walk like me, Marty. Do you want me to go tell your therapists that you're ready now?" Chris spoke slowly, as if to a small child, so my simple mind could understand. I was grateful.

I nodded.

"So I'll tell them that you're gonna start trying hard, you're really gonna do it the way we all know you can? That you really want to get out of this place and come home with us?"

"Come... on... Kwiss," I pleaded. "I... wan... go." Chris seemed to be saying that I had a choice in the matter. But did he mean that if I did everything they asked of me, that I could get out of here?

"How... go?" I began to drool.

"Marty, all you gotta do is pretend like you're riding your bike up a steep hill. It's gonna be hard, but I know you can do it. Just start trying. If it gets hard to do something, don't give up. I never saw you give up before, but now when I watch them ask you to do certain things, you just stop when it gets to be a little hard."

But inside I knew I had not wanted to play their game because I had not understood the object of it—until now.

"If... I... twyy... I... go?"

"Come on, Marty, I know you. You'll be out of this stupid place in no time if you start sucking your gut. Everyone's wondering when the old Marty's going to fire up."

That was all I needed to hear. I was finally realizing that healthy people did not live in hospitals. I would force my way out of this dilemma.

"Juuh... ss... Wa... tchhh." My words did not convey the conviction I wanted them to.

After Chris left, I thought about what he'd said. It seemed like I was finally, slowly awakening from a very heavy sleep.

I realized next that walking would be my pass out of this place. I focused on walking like a man possessed. Chris, who came to see me daily, kept me on track. And Janice was now visiting me regularly and helping me tremendously. If I complained that a particular task that the therapists were asking me to do wasn't helping me to learn how to walk, they would remind me that the therapists knew what they were doing and that I must follow their instructions even though I didn't understand the point. They kept encouraging me to try my best at everything they asked me to do.

I spent most of each day sleeping, maybe eighteen hours or more, but while I was awake I slowly became more oriented and aware. Each day people, places, and things became just a little bit less fuzzy. I felt less and less like I was packaged in foam. I began to sense that there was an "I" to me; that I was an individual, not just this blob of nothingness that was just there. Sounds became more discernible, where before they had all just blended into one tone. For a long time, except for sugary foods, everything tasted like cardboard. That was slowly changing, although the hospital food didn't help much.

I realized that my mind-body connections were badly screwed up. Not only was my right side still paralyzed, but almost no part of my body would do what I told it to do. If I'd been any more aware, the thought of living like that for the rest of my life would have been terrifying. But I had no problem sleeping.

When morning came and I awoke, my actions now had purpose. Chris helped me to increase my workload to four or five short therapy sessions a day. Whether it was learning how to tie my shoes or crawl on a rug, each one completely exhausted me. During my last four weeks of this intensive crash course, I could be found doing one of two things: sleeping in my room or trembling through a therapy session.

Despite my exhaustive days, I always managed to awaken for the hour of joy that my steady stream of nightly visitors brought. Chris worked overtime, night and day, to get me out. The rest of my family, my mother, my father, and my sisters, came by almost every day. And Chris encouraged my friends, other family members, and people from work to visit me. Chris made sure that everyone who came to see me brought laughter and words of encouragement. I don't think I could have gotten better without that support.

One of the secretaries at my firm, Linda, had brought me a small stuffed weasel. She thought it would remind me of the office and how I used to, in her words, "weasel" out of certain jobs by getting her to do them for me.

One day a few weeks later, I tossed it weakly at Rich Milan, whose back was turned to me. Rich had been one of my best friends at college. I looked up to Rich. Strong, tall, and good-looking, he was a winner on many levels. A small-college all-American in track and field, he always had the coolest cars and prettiest girlfriends.

As the weasel bounced off the back of Rich's head, John Tindell called out in his abrasive way. "Hey, look's like he's up to his old tricks. Man, remember when Krieg used to start those mud wars when we were water-skiing?"

"Yeah, Krieg was always starting something." Rich gently tossed the small stuffed object back at me.

I laughed so much my stomach hurt. I was doing a lot better after several weeks of intensive therapy. My motor skills were improving, though my speech was still very ragged. I threw the weasel back again.

"You think you're pretty funny, don't you? Man, you're still the same old crazy Krieg." Rich laughed.

Tindell picked the toy up. "Krieg, I'm tired of tossing this stupid little brown thing around. What is it, a weasel or something?"

"You better watch out, Tindell. He also throws that bandage wrap there, remember?" said Rich.

But John was no longer grinning and his voice had lost its playful tone. "I'll tell you, Krieg, I don't know who thinks you're a weasel, but you know who you remind me of? Rocky, that's who." John set a small blue satin pillow on my bed. It was shaped like a pair of boxing trunks, with the name "Rocky" inscribed in big bold letters across the top.

Tindell had always sounded drunk to me, and his long, surfer-blond hair and casual manner made it hard to take anything he said seriously. But he was serious now. He had been referring to the Sylvester Stallone movie of a year ago about a boxer who fought his way out of the slums. But somehow I couldn't remember it, and my face must have shown it.

"Man, you've seen *Rocky*, haven't you?"

"I don't think Krieg has seen that movie," Rich said. "Come on, Tindell, give the guy a break. He's been stuck in this hospital for a long time."

"It doesn't matter. Krieg, we still think you're a man. You ain't no stupid weasel. I kind of think you're like this Rocky guy. He fights his way out of a pretty bad jam. And that's what we all think you're doing. Right, Milan?"

"You're gonna be back with us in no time, Krieg. We hear you've been hitting it pretty hard. Just don't let up. We're rooting for you," Rich said. Did they realize how much words like that helped me, motivated me, kept me going?

I discovered new ways to push myself, knowing that I was thought of by my peers as a man. Even though I could still barely understand my predicament, the need to prove my manhood drove me as though it were a natural instinct. I was intoxicated by my need to impress these people, to show them they were right about me. I *was* a man.

As I dreamed up new ways to impress the body healers who had been assigned to me, I felt separate from the other therapy patients. I sensed that they were envious of my successes, and I was afraid they would only hold me back. Instead of developing any compassion for them, I began to resent them. In my confused mental state, I did not understand why I was improving and they were not. I reasoned that it was best if I just stayed away from them, since they were probably as retarded as they acted.

Every staring wheelchair patient I passed as my attendant helped me walk slowly down the tiled hallways made me want out even more. I grew even more impatient to leave.

"Kwiss... when... do I get out? How much... more?" I said haltingly to Chris one day.

"Marty, they won't let you out until you can prove you can make it on your own. You've got to show them you can walk, for example, without help," said Chris.

"How?"

"I don't know if they'll let you go if you can only do it on a cane. How 'bout if I ask for you? I don't want you around here much longer, either. I think it's only going to hold you back. You seem like the only guy who's trying around here."

Things began to move faster after I learned how to really talk. The hospital allowed me to leave on weekends to be with my family. This taste of the outside world only compounded my urgent need to break free.

I realized that a wonderful—though confusing—world of color and choice awaited me on the outside. I became increasingly impatient with my predicament. My visits home showed me that I did not have to wait until an attendant was ready before I could relieve myself. I did not have to be strapped to a toilet with an attendant present while using the bathroom.

I now knew that food didn't have to look or taste the same every day. My visits home showed me that the temperature and the pressure of the shower could be regulated, and that I did not have to take one with a group or feel rushed while doing so. These revelations and many others were small, sometimes trivial, but each one was important. Each one made me want to leave the hospital that much sooner.

One day Jake and Paul, two of my bosses at ETEC, visited one afternoon. We talked a short while, then they quickly made it clear why they'd come.

"Marty, everyone tells us that you're doing pretty good. You know, we sure could use you back at the farm—those receivables are really stacking up," said Paul.

They were both tall, though a layer of fat surrounded Paul's soft chin. Paul's work as the company controller had kept him inside, and he had let his body grow flabby. Jake's tan skin and strong muscular body, on the other hand, were products of the gym he belonged to and the sailboat he raced on weekends. He baby-sat his venture capital interest in our fledgling electronics company. I respected them both.

"That's right, Marty. We need you to get on the Siemens account. They like you over there in Germany," Jake added.

Accounting. It seemed like another lifetime. I had forgotten all about it. And now, two powerful authority figures hovered over me in their business suits, demanding that I remember.

"So when you gonna be out of here?" said Paul.

I only knew that I was following Chris's instructions. I did not want to complicate them with a date. That was more than I could handle.

"I... don't... know," I stammered. My reply was more flustered than usual.

"Well, if you don't know, I guess we'll have to hire someone else for your position. Jake and I can't keep covering for you." Paul sounded impatient.

"Marty, just give us some kind of time frame so we can plan around it," Jake suggested.

I looked away. I honestly did not care about work. But I did want to please these two authority figures.

"What do you say, Marty. It's Friday the fourteenth... what about two more weeks, two months, a year... Can you give us some kind of idea?"

My mind was not working very well. I blurted out the first number I remembered. "Two."

"Great," Jake said, and he winked at Paul. "Is that two weeks, two months, or two years? Where you at, tiger?"

"Weeks," I managed to whisper.

"Last Friday of this month. Sounds great! We're gonna hold you to it," Jake said as he and Paul got up to leave.

I nodded. I wanted the pressure to end.

Paul looked at me. "Well, we gotta head back. GC is shipping today. You remember how those guys in engineering are when it comes to costing out things that don't ship. We've gotta keep an eye on them. Good luck, Marty."

I nodded again. A smile crossed my face as I thought about how they were treating me like a big shot.

"Hurry and get out of here, Marty. We've got some big plans for you," said Paul.

"Two weeks, right, Marty?" Jake said. "You almost look like you're ready to go now."

"Two," I grunted, anxious for them to leave. When they did, I sank back in my bed in exhaustion and confusion.

As the days raced by, I began to realize the challenge I

had placed before myself. My guests also reminded me—continuously.

"So you're gonna be out of here by the end of the month? That's great, Marty! Everyone at your office is very excited," Janice said to me.

Janice and Chris covered me in shifts. If Chris was not on hand, Janice was there, watching me with her protective, loving gaze. Blond, petite, and blue-eyed, with a face full of freckles, Janice looked like the classic girl next door. Her bubbly personality provided a perfect complement to her wholesomeness.

"Gooh... " I managed to say.

"Marty, does 'good' mean you're gonna be out in only a few more days?"

I nodded.

After a week had passed, a week which included an entire weekend with my family, all of my friends were talking about how I was entering my last week of therapy.

In the excitement, however, I lost a little bit of my desire to improve. When Friday the fourteenth arrived, the hospital officials decided that I was not yet ready to leave.

"We're sorry, Mr. Krieg, your son is not totally coherent. We cannot release him just yet," Dr. Rollins said to my dad that morning. With the assistance of a cane, I was standing against the wall. They stood on either side of me. Dr. Rollins was overseeing my rehabilitation. We were in the lobby, and the fluorescent lights shone down on the doctor's bald head.

"What happened, Doctor?" My dad asked.

"Well, John, as you know, your boy has made some incredible advances. We've never seen anything like it here before. We're really pleased to see him walking with his cane. But we're concerned about his cognitive skills. For instance, just two days ago he got lost on our elevator. He kept going up and down in it in his wheelchair, and when a nurse finally stopped him, he said he was looking for the third floor. John, you know we only have two floors here." Rollins raised his eyebrows. "Furthermore, there are many fine motor skills he must still reacquire."

"What kinds of things are we talking about?"

"Well... for example, he still can't sign his name."

"Can't he work on something like that at home?"

"We'd also like to see him be able to count change and

fasten a shirt button. There's a whole list of necessary skills he must complete."

"Well... you guys are the experts. Looks like you've got some more work ahead of you, Son." Dad didn't seem too surprised by the doctor's report.

I dropped my head between my arms. Tears welled up in my eyes. My throat clogged up as my body went numb.

"Son, I agree with the doctor. What's another week or two?"

I couldn't take it anymore.

"I'm... not... stay... ing."

My father looked into my eyes for a while, then turned to Rollins. "Doctor, I know my boy. He's pretty stubborn... Do you think he's gonna be any good here staying against his will?"

"Personally, I'd feel a lot better about Marty if you let us keep him a little while longer. I think that he'll be able to build his cognitive abilities by mastering some of the tasks we talked about."

"No... way," I blurted.

"Well then, Marty, let me show your father what I mean. I'll ask you a few simple questions and demonstrate to your dad some of your deficiencies. Does that sound okay with you?"

"Yeh." I was defiant.

"Okay then, can you tell me what color your hair is?"

"Bwown," I exclaimed. No problem.

"Great, Marty. At least you remember what you look like. Sometimes we get people in here who don't even know that we're letting them see themselves when we put them in front of a mirror. Now I'm going to hit you with a little bit tougher one. We're going to see if you even know what's going on around you. What day is today?"

Rollins looked away to the clock. My stomach began to churn. I didn't know.

"I'll give you a hint. We've got a weekend coming up."

I paused, trying to remember the significance of weekends. Calendars and clocks no longer were a part of my life. If other patients were leaving to go home with their families, that meant that the week itself was over and that today was... "Friday!" I proclaimed.

"That's two for two, Marty. You've never let us see such a quick mind before. The last question I'm going to ask you is going to test your memory a little bit. The president of the United States has been around for a couple of years now. Surely you used to see his name in the papers quite a bit. What's his name?"

"Nishon," I blurted.

"No, Marty, we impeached him." Dr. Rollins smiled.

"Ag... new." I continued to be impulsive.

"No, Marty, he made a lot of headlines, probably when you were in college, but that's not it, either. Three strikes and you're out. I'll give you one more chance."

Dad fidgeted as I raced through every archive that I had stored in my mind. My breath hastened as I tried to remember. I knew if he got me on this one, I'd be stuck here. Just as I stopped trying to remember, a press clipping jumped out at me.

"Phoood," I said.

Both of their faces broke out in large grins. Dr. Rollins was surprised, I could tell. "Ford is right. That's great, Marty! Looks like you're not going to let me stump you after all. I guess he's all yours, John. But if Marty is having any difficulties at home, please don't hesitate to call me. We can always readmit him."

"Thanks, Doctor. I can see Marty's got a lot of work ahead of him, but please thank your staff for all the support you gave him. You built a pretty good foundation. So where do we go to sign up for outpatient therapy?"

I was free! My eyes widened in disbelief, and I started to cry. My concentration was starting to slip. I steadied myself against the nearby wall. The lobby and everything in it faded out of focus as I realized that I was escaping this antiseptic hospital full of uniforms and chalky colors. I was returning to the outside world of ever-changing hues and shapes and forms for good. I felt triumphant, and a smile broke across my face.

I would soon find out that it was a lot tougher to make it on the outside.

Chapter 3

COMING HOME

The drive home was a frightening world of glaring stoplights, dashing automobiles, and a bewildering array of signs and buildings. By the time Dad pulled into a strangely familiar cul-de-sac, my mind was dizzy with this new world. The bright morning sun illuminated lawns and driveways dotted with smiling faces and waving hands.

"All right, Marty!" one voice called. "Welcome back," called another. I sat expressionless as Dad looked over at me to see my reaction.

"Don't you recognize any of those people, Marty?"

I didn't answer. "Those are all your neighbors," Dad said as we stopped in front of a brown house. A basketball hoop hovered high above a late-model BMW sedan. "They've all been asking about you... although it's hard to believe they actually missed you and your hot-rodding friends." He smiled and patted my shoulder.

As soon as we stopped, the rest of my family poured out the front door.

"Marty, Marty, Marty, we knew you could do it," Kathy said to me. She was my attractive oldest sister.

"Come on, you kids, let Marty through," Mom said as she cleared a path to the front porch. I hobbled up the steps. By now, the neighbors had also begun to filter over for my homecoming.

"Hey, Jerry, when's Marty gonna be all better?" Mr. Serano asked my mom from the sidewalk.

"He's home, isn't he?" Mom said as she helped me step up onto the porch.

"No, what I want to know is how much longer till he doesn't have to return to the hospital?"

"He's home for good, George," Nancy, my middle sister, volunteered.

"Well, it's up to him... but he still has some outpatient work to do," Mom added as she opened the tattered screen door for me.

I started to slowly walk inside when she asked, "Aren't you going to wave goodbye, Marty?"

The car ride had worn me out. I could barely understand her. "Turn around and wave goodbye, Marty, come on," she implored with her large brown eyes.

I turned around and waved feebly. A sea of faces that looked like one homogeneous glob of smiles looked up at me. Their words of encouragement and congratulation made no sense to me.

I staggered inside and collapsed on the couch in exhaustion. I fell asleep immediately. Several hours later, a bell in the kitchen rang and stopped. Then it rang again. Mom, who always kept a watchful eye on me, noted my perplexed look.

"I'll bet Marty would like to talk on the telephone," she said just as my sister answered it. "Is that for Marty?"

"It's Uncle Danny for Marty," Karen called.

"Here, Chris, you take one side and I'll take the other," Dad said as both of them picked me up and brought me to the kitchen wall phone.

"Chum Choy, you made it," the voice on the other end said as Dad helped me hold the receiver up to my ear.

My eyes revealed the surprise that I felt. The whole telephone experience seemed like magic to me. I didn't know what to do next.

"Go ahead, say something, Marty," said Kathy.

"Who... is... dis?" I asked. My family laughed.

"It's Uncle Dan, Marty, remember me?"

"I... thiiink... tho." Dan and I had shared a lot over the years. Even though he was my uncle, he was my age and we had grown up together making forts, playing sports, and stealing fruit from the neighborhood trees where he lived in Alameda, California. He had decided to call me Chum Choy on a motorcycle trip we had made to Canada; I had introduced him as Gum Chewy to a girl he was trying to impress.

"You going to be riding your 550 pretty soon?" It took me a few seconds to realize he was talking about my motorcycle.

"Where... is... it?"

"It should still be parked in your garage. Your BMW's still there, I saw it just a couple of days ago when I drove by."

"Oh... " I didn't really care about either. Unable to

maintain the needed concentration to hold a conversation, I handed the phone back to my brother without even saying goodbye to Dan.

"What do you say we all clear out of here and let Marty get some rest," Mom said gently. "He gets tired easily, and all the people and all the excitement today have been a little bit too much for him."

For the rest of the day and night I slept. The next two weeks I slept most of the day, just as I had in the hospital. It was still hard to focus my eyes, and I was still in a haze when I was awake. I tried to work on the simplest things, but even basic skills eluded me. Brushing my teeth was a major chore—I always cut my lips and gums with the brush. I would stab my tongue with my fork. Tying my shoes, shaving, putting my watch on, fastening buttons—nothing requiring basic motor skills came easy. I wasn't making much progress, though my paralyzed right side was slowly responding.

A couple of weeks after I got home I began to make infrequent appearances at work. I wasn't capable of much of anything besides showing up—I think I was more of an inspirational tool than anything else—but I was an intermittent presence at ETEC for the next several months, mostly in the afternoons.

One morning I awoke to a furry hairball of energy that exploded into my room.

"Alex! Come on, Alex, leave Marty alone," Chris called frantically as he tried to keep our dog away from me.

I could not defend myself as Alex, the chow chow that Chris and I owned, slobbered and grunted all over me. His happy, carefree manner was appealing to me. I wondered how I could get that way.

"Sorry, Marty," Chris said as he finally separated the two of us. "Hey, Janice has to work today so she can't come over and watch you, but Nancy's coming over with Ben."

Just as they had in the hospital, Chris and Janice would still take turns watching me. Janice now worked as a waitress at night and took care of me during the day. Chris, who worked during the days delivering lumber, watched me at night.

"Nancy?" I asked. I was learning how to inflect my words.

"Yeah, you remember your sister, don't you? Well, she's bringing Little Ben, so you can have a good laugh watching him like you always do. She'll be here any minute but I gotta go. Catch you tonight." Chris grabbed his lunch pail and dashed out the front door.

When Nancy arrived I found out who Little Ben was—Nancy's young son. I soon realized that I felt challenged by him. Both of us had to learn a lot of the same basic living skills: walking, eating, proper use of the bathroom, balancing one's self, and command of fine motor skills. Even though I laughed at him as he teetered and swayed, a part of me dimly knew that I wasn't much more advanced.

Later on that day, as I let Ben amuse me, a familiar voice interrupted us from the front porch.

"God, Krieg," It was Rich Milan. His voice called through the screen door. "You ain't gonna get better that way."

"Come on in, Rich," Nancy called from the kitchen, where she was fixing me lunch. Rich came in and sat down on the couch and watched us on the floor.

"Is that what Marty does for therapy now? What's your little boy's name?"

"That's Benjamin," Nancy yelled.

"Well, I'll tell ya, Marty ain't gonna get any better watching little Benjamin play," Rich said. "Is that all you've been doing for the last two weeks, Krieg, is just laying around? Man, I thought you'd be out on your basketball court shooting hoops by now."

"They tol... me... rest... is part... of my... heal... ing," I rationalized in my whisper-like voice.

"Well, I don't think they meant all the time."

"I'm... doin... some... things."

"Like what, Krieg?"

I couldn't think of an answer. "What... kind of... ex... er... cises... do you re... com... mend?"

"Aren't you doing anything to help you get around better?"

"Like... wha?"

He watched me struggle to hold my head up just so that I could look at him, then said, "Krieg, you don't just need exercises, you need professional help, therapy."

Nancy poked her head in. "Mom has him signed up for outpatient therapy over at Fairmont. He's on the waiting list right now. C'mon, Rich, give him a break. He just got out of the hospital."

"I know—two weeks ago. That's not the way it works,

Nancy. You can't let him get into the habit of resting on his laurels. He's gotta keep working as hard now as he did to get out of that place. This is no time to let up. He's probably got the hardest part still ahead of him."

"Why don't you put yourself in his shoes, Rich? I think he's doing pretty damn good. I don't think you could have done what he's done. You know, you think because you're this big famous track star that everyone's supposed to be at your level or else they're lazy. Just let up on him." Nancy was irritated. I just sat on the floor with Ben and watched them, only dimly comprehending what they were discussing.

Rich ignored her. "Krieg, I'll bet Chu can help you."

"Chu?"

"Yeah, Don Chu, don't you remember? He's that trainer up at Cal State. Don't you remember our track team? Chu had all those guys breaking conference records."

"Yeah... " I slowly nodded.

"Well, he's starting this sports therapy practice over in Castro Valley and he usually only works with injured athletes, like world-class high jumpers and stuff. But I'll see if I can talk him into helping you."

A light went on in my head.

"Rich... can you... please... see if... you can?"

"I'll see what I can do. You need help, Krieg, and this stuff—" he motioned toward Ben and me—"is just not gonna cut it." With that he walked out of the house.

Sleep proved difficult over the next few days as I imagined what it would be like to be treated like an injured athlete. Being thought of that way inspired me a lot more than being considered a cripple. But despite the fact that Rich recognized the urgency of my dilemma, he didn't get back to me quickly. Each day that passed felt like a lifetime. I began to panic after a few days.

"Hey, Nancy... can you call Rich?"

"Marty, I just called him twenty minutes ago. You've been asking me to call him every five minutes for the last three days. You should know your friend by now. He comes and goes when he feels like it. He'll show up. I'm getting tired of listening to his phone ring, Marty, but he'll be here."

That afternoon I heard a car screeching to a halt at the curb in front of the house. It was Rich. Three days had passed.

Rich bounded into the house. "Hop in the car, Krieg. Chu wants to take a look at you up at the college."

A half-hour later we pulled up to school. I was on the verge of fainting. The sensation of driving in Rich's little Volkswagen Bug had induced several dizzy spells. The walk from the parking lot to the gymnasium was an additional challenge to my continued consciousness. The bodies scurrying about in every direction overloaded my senses, and the bright sun was blinding. It was quite a switch from the calm interior of my house.

Rich started up the sidewalk, then turned and waited for me as I struggled on my cane to keep up.

"God, Krieg, I remember when you used to run up and down these walkways backwards. You're doing great, though. Let's stop for a minute and rest." We sat down on a concrete bench under a newly planted tree.

We finally made it to the air-conditioned building. An ocean of tiled floors and endless hallways led us to the gymnastics area, where Don was teaching a class. We entered the room. Rich pointed out Don across the room. He was leaning against the trampoline supports. Don was a big guy in his mid-thirties with a sunny demeanor that seemed almost childlike. He was robust and cheerful, and his dark hair parted at the side complemented his tan skin. He radiated warmth and vitality.

Thoroughbred athletes jumped and bounced throughout the room as Don Chu looked on approvingly. His reputation extended far beyond Cal State Hayward. A trainer at the 1976 Olympic trials, he had worked with many premier athletes and professional sports teams. He had a Ph.D. from Stanford, and he had authored many books and articles in the field of sports therapy. He was even known as the father of plyometrics, a new athletic training regimen that was collecting momentum all around the world. Don Chu was famous, and in my weakened state I felt tremendously intimidated. What would he care about an insignificant shrimp like me?

I felt near collapse, but I tried my best to look like an injured athlete as I slumped against the mirrored wall. The room cartwheeled inside of my head as I tried to focus on one activity. The clothes hanging loosely from my gaunt, pale body belied the image I was trying to convey.

Don walked right over. "So… Rich tells me you were in a car accident."

I nodded. I felt dizzy, and my eyes were glassy.

He appraised me. I just knew I wouldn't measure up. Then he said, "Do you think you can come by my Castro Valley office Monday so I can take a better look?"

I perked up a bit at that. "I think... tho," I said, trying to hold myself up straighter.

"Well, if transportation's a problem, maybe we can get Rich to bring you in."

Just then, a volleyball bounced off Don's clipboard, knocking his pen to the ground. It startled me. I was terrified that the magic spell would be broken, and he would change his mind. The room grew quiet.

Don broke the tension. "Come on... can't you guys see that I'm not playing?"

Everyone laughed. The noise level rose again.

"I'll make sure he has a ride," Rich said.

"Great. We'll take a look at you first thing Monday morning, okay Marty?" Don waited for my reaction.

"Oh... kay," I said, trying to conceal my excitement.

Moments later we were back in Rich's car, whizzing through traffic. "God, Krieg, am I making you sick or something?" Rich said as he zipped in and out of traffic on the way home. I was hanging my head out of the window. His car always smelled like oil, and I was badly in need of fresh air. I did not answer.

"I remember when you used to scare the shit out of me in that little Spitfire of yours. You were always showing off how great your car handled corners."

A moving van finally forced Rich to slow down.

"I don't know why they let these damn trucks go so slow. There oughta be a speed limit for slow vehicles, too. Hey, Krieg, I'm excited for you. You got Chu on your side now. Aren't you excited?"

"Yeah."

I was barely able to comprehend the significance of the day's events, and I was exhausted to the point of incoherence. I didn't even say goodbye or thanks when he let me off. I just let Janice meet me at the door and guide me to my bedroom. I slept straight through till the next day.

"How would you like to go shopping for some new tennis shoes today, Marty?" Janice's smiling face the next day welcomed me to a bright, sunny morning. "How about if we eat some breakfast, then I'll drive you over to Southland? They've got some pretty good sales at Penney's."

"Shoes?"

"Haven't you noticed that you've only got one pair of shoes? They couldn't get both pairs out of the car, it was so smashed. You also lost your toolbox the same way."

"Smashed?"

"Your mom says that they could barely get you out the back window. Maybe they'll also have some nice shirts you can wear. You're going back to see your friends at work and you want to look nice, don't you? You got blood stains on some of your best clothes, Marty. But you've got lots of money in your checking account, so let's go get you looking good again."

Like everything that was not hospital white, the department store overloaded my senses. My dull mind simply could not process so much information. While bright colors and signs begged for my attention, the music, bells, and voices that blared from high-above speakers surrounded me in a three-dimensional nightmare. The fluorescent lights made me feel vulnerable, exposed. They demanded that I summon every last ounce of strength just to remain standing. As people busily scurried about on one screen of this surreal multiplex, a slow-motion movie seemed to be playing on another. It showed stationary people disappearing into the ceiling and others emerging, all on moving metal staircases. It was all new and strange and bewildering.

We made it to the shoe department, where the different colors and styles and shapes confused me even more. Janice handled the purchase for me as I leered in awe at the busy throngs. They all seemed to know what they were doing and where they were going.

"You want that pair, Marty? Now you have to pay for it. Here, I brought your checkbook." We followed the clerk to the cash register.

"That'll be $29.97, sir," the clerk said.

"I'll fill in everything but your signature, Marty. I can't do that," Janice entered the date and the amount. "I can tie your shoes for you and help you fasten your shirt buttons, but I can't sign your name, you have to do that. Here's a pen."

I fidgeted as I nervously held the writing instrument in my hand. All eyes were on me.

"Go ahead, Marty, like you always used to, just sign here," Janice said, pointing to the appropriate place on my check.

My pen erratically skipped off the paper, leaving only a line.

"That's okay, Marty, try another one," Janice said. The clerk curiously looked on.

Once again, my trembling hand could not control the pen's movement. The result was no better.

"He was in a car accident. He was paralyzed and he doesn't have real good control of some things," Janice said in a low voice. "Can I sign for him?"

I knew that it must be clear that something was not right with me, but I didn't want to rely on that excuse. But I didn't have the vocabulary to tell Janice how I felt, so I just kept quiet. I was upset and embarrassed.

"Let me ask my manager," answered the young clerk.

While we waited for the manager, the clerk said, "Paralyzed, huh? I'll bet you've had to work on some stuff."

I nodded. I tried not to smile. I had endured a lot of the pain I had felt back in the hospital by grinding my front teeth together, and I was overly conscious of how pointy my teeth were.

"He really has come a long way," said Janice. "It's just that now we get to work on all the little things, like using keys to open doors and counting change and putting on a watch. Marty's not used to having to work at anything. It always used to come so easy for him."

"Yeah... we just take so many things for granted, don't we?" returned the insightful clerk.

When the manager walked up, Janice convinced him that the hospital had let me sign my way out with an "X". He granted us the same privilege.

Something as simple as signing my own name had become a major production. The event had tired me.

"Janice... let's go."

"Don't you want to look at anything else?"

"Just want... to sleep." I felt completely drained.

We drove home. I spent most of the weekend sleeping in preparation for my first session with Don Chu. My fears became magnified. If I couldn't do a simple thing like sign my own name, how could I do any of the things Don would expect from me?

Monday morning finally came. It would prove to be the beginning of my new life.

Chapter 4

LEARNING TO WALK

"Marty, I think Rich is at the door," Janice yelled from the shower. It was early the next morning, and I was ready to go.

"Come in," I said as loud as I could. The knocking continued. He hadn't heard my feeble voice. As I slowly walked to the door, I tried again. "Come in."

The doorknob rotated. Click, click. "It's locked," yelled Rich. "Hurry up, Krieg. We've got to make it to Chu's, then I've got to get back to my class."

Janice ran by me in a towel and opened the door.

"Hi, Janice. Nice outfit. God, Krieg, you take forever," Rich said, bursting in. He wore running shorts, a T-shirt, and running sneakers, his standard uniform. "You're like an old man." He walked into the kitchen. "Got any clean glasses around here? I'm thirsty." I could hear him rummaging through the cabinets.

"What time are you guys gonna be back?" Janice asked from the bedroom. "Marty can't unlock the door by himself, so I'll have to know when someone should be here in case my lab runs late." Janice was taking a few classes at the local junior college in addition to working as a waitress.

"I'll pick him up after my class. We'll probably be back around noon." He slammed his empty water glass down and walked into the front room. "Let's go, Krieg."

"Wait a minute, Rich, I can pick him up then. Is that the place over in Castro Village?"

"You want to? It's on the Santa Maria side. It's called—"

"I know, I know, Ather Sports Injury Clinic, that's all Marty's been talking about."

Rich hustled me into his car and we roared away. I knew I was making progress when I began to recognize certain buildings and other landmarks on the way to Don's office. Still, our short three-mile jaunt through town felt like a roller-coaster ride. To keep from getting sick, I focused on the scenery instead of the blur of cars, people, and lights zooming by us in every direction.

"Janice'll be here in an hour," Rich said as he left me off at the sidewalk in front of Chu's office. He pulled away from the curb, then stopped and leaned out the window. "Krieg... good luck. Don't let me down."

As Rich sped off, I turned and studied the small sign which hung above the door. The words "Ather Sports Injury Clinic" surrounded an athlete confidently soaring over a hurdle. With the many obstacles that lay before me, seeing that boosted my confidence.

I braced myself as best I could and tried to open the door. But every time I tried to get my body inside the screen door, it slammed shut. Not a good way to start the day.

"Kim, I think Marty's trying to get inside. Can you go help him with the door?" It was Don's voice. A moment later a slim, healthy young woman with long light-brown hair smiled as she let me in.

Some athlete, I thought, as I sheepishly looked around the clinic. The room was about twenty by fifteen feet, with a little office in the corner. There were only a few windows near the glass door. Sports posters covered the walls, and cardboard boxes stuffed with gym shorts lined the counter that ran along one wall. A weight scale stood alongside a medicine ball and chrome-plated weights, and there were several different weight machines and therapy tables scattered around the room. I watched Kim move around the room from one patient to another with an efficient elegance.

In a while Don came over to where I leaned on my cane.

"Have a seat, Marty," Don said. "All we're going to do today is see what we're working with, so you can just relax. Then we'll figure out a schedule for you."

Kim joined us as he spoke. It turned out that Kim was Don's assistant and one of his track and field stars.

"Now, Marty," Don began, "I'm going to conduct a little examination." He reached for a clipboard with his powerful arm. "We've got to know as much as we can before we put you on a program."

For the next half-hour Don probed and measured and turned and twisted and bent. I tried to force my body to respond in the way that I thought an injured athlete's would. I prayed that I'd responded correctly.

Don was all business during the exam. But when it was over, he smiled. "Well, essentially you're a right hemiplegic, but it looks like you're all hooked up, big guy. That's a good sign. We got some work ahead of us, though. I want to start on your legs."

I could hardly control my breathing. It sounded like he was treating me like one of his athletes already.

Don outlined the basics of what my regimen would be, and what he hoped it would do. When he finished, he put down his clipboard and looked at me. "But Marty, you're the one who decides what's gonna happen to you."

"Me?"

"That's right. It's all gonna have to be up to you. I can give you the direction, but in the end, you're gonna be running the show. If you're ready to really work at it, I'll see you in here starting tomorrow, five days a week, three hours a day. Sound like a good plan?"

My heart began to beat faster. "Yeah," I answered, already short of breath.

Don turned to Kim. "I'm going to need you to ask his mom or dad to call me so we can get the times all set up. We'll also need to figure out the transportation and get all the insurance forms filled out. Oh, and Kim, can you see if Marty's ride is here yet?"

"I think I just heard someone pull up," answered Kim. She helped me to the door.

"Bye," I called to Don as I walked out.

"Don's gonna... take me," I tried to shout to Janice as she approached me on the sidewalk.

"Say again, Marty?" Janice placed her arms around me.

"Don's... gonna... take... me." I formed the words as clearly as I could. A tear ran down Janice's cheek.

"That's great, Marty. I knew you could do it. But you know what that means, don't you?"

"What?"

"It means you can't just lay around by the wall heater anymore. You're setting yourself up for some pretty big challenges all over again. You're sure you don't want a little more rest? I mean, I love you the way you are. You don't have to do anything to win my heart, you know."

"Any... thing to be normal," I said.

Janice said nothing, but another tear trickled down her face. She was realizing that this child of a man she had fallen in love with was turning into a machine with little time to consider anyone else's feelings.

As I entered Don's clinic the following morning, I recalled to myself how easy life was before the accident. In the past, if I had wanted to go somewhere, I didn't have to wait until someone was ready to take me. Logistical discussions about the availability of bathrooms, how high a curb was, or the number of steps which separated me from an entrance never preceded any of the trips I took.

All of the attention that my family and Janice focused on my mobility, however, strengthened my resolve to make the most of my time with Don. Those three hours every day became the event I built my whole day around. Nothing else mattered to me.

My first few days at the clinic were filled with apprehension. Could I perform well enough? Would they send me home because I was not improving fast enough? What if they found out I was not an athlete? These were just a few of the worries that had already started that morning.

"Well, well. You're right on time, champ. You ready to hit it a hundred percent today?" Don's confident voice greeted me, and Kim directed me to a therapy table.

"I'll be with ya in a second, champ," Don said. He was busy with another patient, so Kim began the torture-like warm-ups that I would come to know so well.

Lightly resting her fingertip on my wrist, she said, "Okay, Marty, I want you to touch your waist, so you'll be taking your arm across your body like this." She showed me the movement. "We're going to be working with your range of motion on this one."

"Okay," I reached for my waist as hard as I could. My body trembled. My arm quivered as it slowly crossed my body. My shoulder felt like it was going to explode out of its socket. The veins in my neck bulged.

I completed the movement. "Great job, Marty. We're gonna rest for a little bit and then we'll hit it again."

Wasn't that good enough, I wondered? And what did she mean by "'we?" I was doing all the work. But I kept quiet.

After several such repetitions, I couldn't even feel my arm. The pain had crossed over into numbness. Kim kept pushing me. "Come on, Marty, don't let up. Drive it."

Finally the phone rang and I got a rest. As Kim talked, I wondered how much more I could have pushed myself.

Don had explained to me that in the world of therapy, tomorrow does not exist—only today. If I didn't give my all every day, I would not improve. Even though my forehead and eyebrows were already wet with perspiration, I knew in my gut that there was an untapped reserve I was yet to discover.

Don finished with his other patient and came over. "Okay, Marty," he said, taking over for Kim, "I want you to turn on your side and push out with your arm just like this." Don showed me as he spoke. "And Kim, I want you to hold right here so that he doesn't cheat with his legs."

Oh God, I thought, two against one. "All right, Marty. We're gonna do this ten times and then we'll give you a rest," said Don.

I got weaker with each try, but I kept pushing... eight, nine, ten. Feeling as hard as I could for the right muscle group to use, I closed my eyes. My body trembled and shook. After a while I didn't even know if I was moving the right body part. My body went limp.

I would quickly grow to love such torture and look forward to it in a perverse way. Every new day of it meant I was improving. Each session became an event that I psyched myself up for long beforehand. Each appointment occupied my every thought as I mentally prepared myself to perform beyond any of the limits I had set for myself.

After a short break, they returned for more. "Okay, let's do it on the reverse side," Don said. And so it continued for ten more repetitions before we went on to another excruciating exercise, then another, then another, each involving a different muscle group. Some of the exercises were followed by a half-hour of electrical stimulation of certain muscles.

I knew I was pushing hard enough when my eyes wanted to explode out of their sockets and my chin and neck felt like they were fused together. But I also knew that I had to keep setting higher and higher limits of pain for myself. Soon I was grimacing and groaning loudly, not caring what Don or Kim or the other patients thought.

After the session was over, I was beyond exhausted. It was the hardest, most painful workout I'd ever experienced. But I was happy.

"How much looonger... do you... thiink... it will... take before I'm normal... again?" I asked Don between breaths.

"I'm not sure what you mean, exactly. Everyone has a different interpretation for that word."

"Well, how... long... till I can be... like you guys?" Each word was slow and deliberate.

Both Don and Kim laughed. "Is that what you call normal?" Kim teased.

"How... long till I can... do things... like I used to?"

Kim sensed how real my concern was and excused herself. Like a father, Don guided me to his tiny office and sat me down.

"Marty, all I know is that you've got to be willing to give it some time. You're doing really great, but I have no idea what goes on up there," he said, pointing to my head. "About all I can say is that it's up to you. Sure, I can compare your progress to date and project where that rate will put you in two weeks, two months, or two years. But, Marty, it all begins and ends with you. How bad do you want it, big guy?"

I leaned closer.

"You know, Marty, I can say one thing and what actually happens can either far exceed your expectations or fall way short. I don't want to tell you something which I'm not really clear on, and you don't want me to mislead you, do you?"

"Then... it's up... to me?"

"You said it, big guy." Somehow, Don's honest pep talk justified the pain.

Because of Don's work at the college, there was a steady stream of athletes throughout the day. Big, strong, and carefree, they were a visual incentive to push myself even harder. I wanted to be able to move my body like them, to walk like them. I felt improvements, but they weren't coming fast enough. Little things still frustrated me.

I still couldn't sign my name. Sometime in December, after we had shifted the emphasis of the exercises to my upper body, I looked at Don. "Hey Don... can you... help me... make... my... signature?"

"Hmm. I'm not an occupational therapist, but I'm sure we can figure that one out. Let's give it a shot.

"What we've got to do is control and direct your motion. How 'bout if I provide resistance and... hey, Kim, can you come over here with a couple pieces of scratch paper?"

"What are we going to do?" Kim asked as she joined us. "Marty's going to draw a circle while I guide his hand through the motion, and I need you to hold the paper down. Ready, Marty?"

I nodded. Thinking circle as hard as I could, the spastic movement that my hand produced tore a hole in the paper.

"That's okay, Marty, concentrate a little harder this time."

I tried again. This time my nervous trembling broke the pencil.

"This is… the worst," I whispered. I felt my eyes tear up.

"You're doing great, Marty. Kim, can you grab us a couple of pens and some more paper?"

As she went off in search of supplies, Don said, "It's this fine-tuning stuff that's not going to give you the kind of results that you've gotten accustomed to, Marty. But you've got to work just as hard. Maybe harder. You can't let up on the little things. They may not seem all that important but I guarantee you they are. If you have the patience to make it through the frustration they cause you, they'll make every challenge you take on seem a little bit easier. They're just going to take a little more time, that's all. Now let's try again."

From circles, we moved on to the alphabet. Each day Don gave me more homework. Besides squeezing tennis balls, doing toe raises, or performing some of the many other exercises that Don prescribed for me to do on my own, I now had to practice drawing letters. I practiced on kindergarten paper—the kind designed for beginning writers, with wide columns divided by broken lines so that beginners can gauge letter size correctly.

Simple conversations still challenged me. People had to stand very close just to hear me.

"What… can I… do… to talk… louder?" I knew Don could help me here, too.

Don scratched his head and thought for a few minutes before answering.

"That's your wind. After we get your legs back you can start placing some demands on your cardiovascular system. That one's gonna take some time, but you'll be there."

That sounded strange coming from Don. I was tired of hearing how time would heal me. Everyone else talked that way about my dilemma, but not Don. He had to know a way to do it now.

"But I'm tired of never being heard."

"How 'bout yelling?" Don offered.

"How?"

"Go out on your street and yell at the top of your voice. Do it as loud as you can. You need to concentrate on your wind. I know, have your brother or your girlfriend take you up to Cal State. Go over to the stadium and walk up and down the bleachers while you're yelling."

"What do I yell?"

"Anything. Call your dog."

I hung on to his every word. Somehow Don could figure out a way to conquer any problem, and I had quickly come to rely on him to help me with the countless problems I faced. In my still simple mind he had come to be a hero.

There were others who also thought of Don as something of a miracle man. He had raised several athletes to national recognition from a relatively obscure college campus that did not even award sports scholarships. According to Rich, Don was able to scientifically enable high jumpers, his specialty, to consistently realize their full potential. Several of his college stars had jumped against the best in world competitions. And I worked among them. It was inspiring.

Don even convinced me that I could be like them. On one occasion, after I had again asked Don if I could ever be normal again, he said, "Marty, if you keep pushing like you've been pushing... well, all I can say is that you're gonna be healthier than anyone I know."

"You sure?"

"Sure I'm sure. You're definitely performing at a world-class level."

My eyes grew large. Whether Don's words were true or not, they would become my mantra.

After a few weeks, when he knew he had my confidence, Don offered to replace my crutch. "I'll tell ya, Marty, if we're going to get you to the top, we've got to get you off that thing," he said as he pointed to the walking aid I went everywhere with. It had become a third leg, and the thought of losing it was a shock. "You're becoming too dependent on it."

Almost as suddenly as I had felt like a superman, I felt betrayed. My stomach began to ache. *I'd like to see him do what I'm doing without a cane,* I thought. Then I caught myself. I knew that Don wanted the best for me. Even if his words sounded cruel, I knew they must be for my own good. My jaw tightened.

"Dependent?"

"That's right," Don said with a smile. "You don't know what I mean, since you've never tried to function without a cane. Just try it. Take a couple of steps."

"How?" I said, as I propped myself against the wall. Wasn't this awfully sudden?

"Come on, Marty. Just put one foot in front of the other, only leave the cane there against the wall. Kim and I will catch you if you fall."

I propped the cane against the wall next to me. The fifteen feet between me and the opposite wall looked as wide as the Grand Canyon. I took a deep breath, then reached out with my right foot. The room began to swirl and gyrate. I felt dizzy. Just as I began to fall, Don caught me.

"Great try, big guy, but did you have a goal?" He helped me lean against one of his therapy tables.

"A goal?" I said as I caught my breath. I felt like I'd just finished a hundred-yard dash.

"That's right, Marty. If you don't know where you're going, how're you gonna get there? You see, your body doesn't operate on automatic anymore. You can't just get up and walk for the sake of walking like you used to. What you've got to do is pick out a spot on the wall or something, focus on it, and not let anything else distract you. Let your goal pull you to it. Then, after a while, you can start increasing your distances, and in a while walking will become automatic again."

"Which spot?"

Walking over to the wall on the other side of the room, Don inserted a red push pin into the wall. "How's that? Okay, let's hit it again, big guy. Don't worry, we'll be on both sides of you and we'll catch you if you start falling. Just do it."

I took a breath and pushed myself away from the table. Fixing my gaze on the red push pin all of fifteen feet away, I summoned all of my available strength and will. Unlike the times back in the hospital when I had tried to walk without a cane, I refused to picture myself collapsing. Instead of seeing nurses or friends rushing to my aid, all I saw was the pin. And all I heard was encouragement from Don and Kim.

Once again, I reached out with my foot. I was wobbly, but after a while I forced the other foot to follow. Unlike the last time, I let go and allowed the momentum of each shaky step to carry me to the pin. I felt like a stick figure, and I remembered little Benjamin's first faltering steps. My body jerked and lurched as my goal grew closer and closer. Every step seemed like a mountain. Every time I felt my body sway sideways, I concentrated even harder on my goal. I felt like an acrobat balancing on a precarious cable high above the ground. As I neared the wall, the voices grew louder. After an eternity, I took a final step and fell forward toward the wall. Don and Kim grabbed me on either side.

"All right, Marty!" Don cheered. He gave me a bear hug.

"That was great, Marty. Pretty soon you're gonna be running. I'm so proud of you," added Kim.

At first, I didn't know what to say. The smile slowly working its way across my face gave way to a feeling of jubilation as I reached out to slap Don's outstretched hand.

Don had given me the confidence to see what I was capable of. He had given me the courage that I would need to carry me over the many obstacles ahead. My journey across those fifteen feet would be an inspiration for a long time to come.

"Marty, now I want you to start walking without that cane. Whenever your judgment tells you that you'll be safe, I want you to walk without it."

After an afternoon of therapy, I usually left the clinic barely able to control my weary body. Today, though, I went out to the parking lot feeling rejuvenated and alive.

"So how'd it go today, Marty?" Janice asked, just as she always did. She started up the car.

"I... wearned... how to walk."

"What do you mean, Marty?" Her voice always had a smile in it.

"Wifout... a cane!"

"All right, Marty, now I can take you to the beach like I promised. Wait till I tell Bob and Jeff. They're planning this big beach party for you, too. Everyone's gonna be there."

"Don says... I got to... pwactice."

"That's all right, Marty. It's a start. You'll be ready in no time."

When I began walking without a cane, I always made sure I was near a wall so I could have something to hold onto in case I should falter. I did my best to avoid crowds. And I always sought out a goal. If I rounded a corner, I made sure to readjust my sights. It slowly got easier and easier.

From walking without a cane, I advanced to jumping. Mastering that, I moved to a metal folding chair; Don helped me with my balance as I stepped up and down on it. By the time I started to learn how to hop on one foot, I wanted to be able to run.

Several weeks later, I ran across the carpeted floor of Don's clinic. Soon, I was running on the sidewalk in front of my house. I wanted to run around the block. I ran from one telephone pole to the next, and after a brief rest at each, I made it.

But I wanted more. I went to sleep and woke up every day with one thought on my mind. I wanted to run a mile without stopping. I talked about it. I dreamed about it. I was obsessed with it. Finally, as my treatments at the clinic grew more and more infrequent, I decided to try it.

Early one morning about four months after my first visit to Don, Janice and I drove over to the nearby Tennyson High School track. While Janice watched from the bleachers, I began working my way around the quarter-mile track. I focused on a different tree or shrub every time the dirt track curved. I limped along at a snail's pace, but I did not stop. The early morning air supercharged my lungs, and my body ached and hurt as it pounded against the hard soil.

Nearly an hour later, I finished my fourth and final lap. I staggered across the finish line that Janice had etched into the dirt for me and into her arms. It felt like I'd just finished a marathon.

"You did it, Marty, you did it. Just like you said you would!" she said as she hugged me. "I'm so proud of you."

I could hardly breathe, much less speak. "How'd I... look," I gasped.

"You looked great." Janice guided me to the nearby stands. Her eyes were wet. "You've come a long way, Marty." There was an odd tone in her voice.

Looking out onto the playing field inside the track, I knew what she meant. I really had come a long way since the accident. And then I realized that somewhere along the way, in my insatiable, self-centered quest to reach the goals that symbolized "normal" for me, I had lost Janice. But I was so single-minded that I didn't care. I didn't have any extra time for anybody else. I was too busy reclaiming my life. Just that was enough for my simple mind.

I could not look back if I was going to reach the big goal that Don had built far ahead of me. I wanted to be healthier than anyone he knew, and both Don and Janice had done as much as they could to get me there.

The car wreck had robbed me of sensitivity to anyone else's needs. Chris had left the house not long before. Like many of my friends, he hadn't been able to put up with me anymore. When Janice moved out a short while later, I was truly on my own.

Chapter 5

ALONE

I had stopped going to Don Chu's in April. Over the past three or four months, he had been my guru, and to a certain extent, he still was. He had helped bring me back into the world both physically and mentally, and he had boosted my confidence tremendously. He had given me the tools, and told me I could make it. But after three months of seeing him once or twice a week, I had decided that I had to do the rest myself. Don had given me a big bear hug and told me that he'd always be there for me. I got pretty emotional, and I left Don's clinic for the last time in tears.

"You hear Janice finally left Krieg?" asked Bob.

"I was wondering how long she'd last. Man, Krieg is so weird ever since his accident," said Jeff. "Hey, when's that waitress coming back with our drinks?"

"Yeah, you get hit on the head, you get better, what's the big deal? Krieg just won't let it go, though. He told Milan the other day that he needs time to work on himself. All of a sudden it's like, here we are his friends, and we get his ass out of the hospital, and now he's too good for us. Hell with that guy."

"Hey, check it out." Bob's attention shifted to two attractive young women who stood on the other side of the dance floor. "Which one do you want?"

"Forget 'em, Beaudry. They're with the band." Jeff performed as a drummer with many of the area musicians and knew a lot about their social circles.

"But she was looking at me. C'mon, let's score."

"Man, you always think chicks are looking at you. Besides, that one with the red hair is with the bouncer."

"Oh well, I tried. Krieg would have talked to 'em. I'll say that much for him. He had nerve."

"Yeah, but he would have found out the same thing. It's

too bad. I think he actually likes being weird. No one can stand to be around him anymore. All he talks about is his accident. You ever see him when he cries now? He's like a little kid." Jeff scrunched his face up and they both laughed.

"Yeah, how about some consistency? Not Krieg—he's either crying or he's so happy he's flying through the roof. It'd be different if he were just down all the time, then we'd know what to expect. I think that's why they fired him. You know that Melanie chick he worked with at ETEC?"

"The one Krieg was seeing with the big—?"

"Yeah, that one. I saw her over at Long's the other day, and she was saying he was a behavior problem. She said they were all excited to have him back and they gave him a secretary to record his phone conversations and everything and then he starts getting all emotional about everything."

"Wasn't he still just working part-time?"

"Nah, he just got back to full, and she said they didn't mind that he wasn't very productive. He was just—I think she used the word—disruptive."

"Same old Krieg, always causing shit. You've got to admit," said Jeff, "you're probably missing the old Marty. Remember when he used to bark at people that were walking on the sidewalk?"

"Yeah, he was fun. Remember all those times when he'd see an old guy on the sidewalk and he'd yell 'Dad'? And did you ever notice how he never did stuff like that in his own car? He always made everyone else feel like their cars were marked."

"And now he wants us to call him Martin. Screw that shit."

"Who had the Coors here," interrupted the waitress.

"That's his. Hey, when are all the women going to start getting here?"

"There's lots of pretty girls here," she said, looking around the dimly lit dance floor. She gave him his change and left.

They both watched her walk away. "Yeah, and they're all sitting with guys," muttered Jeff.

"Well, the new Martin really blew it for Chris and me last weekend," said Bob.

"What'd he do this time?"

"Oh man, we're walking along and there's these foxy

chicks we're following over on Union Street and they'd been smiling at me and Chris all night long at this disco."

"What, that place you're always talking about over there in the city?"

"Yeah, you know, the 2020. We're all going back to our cars and all of a sudden, Marty blurts out, 'Hey, where you ladies going?' and these chicks took off running. I shit you not. Running. I couldn't believe it. I know me and Chris could have scored. These chicks were ready, man." Bob shook his head in disgust.

"I think Marty thinks he's still got his old charm. Remember all those girls he turned you on to?" Jeff took off his glasses and started cleaning them.

"Lim, when you gonna put some new tape on those glasses? No, one look at those weird, glassy eyes and that droopy face and I think you'd take off running if you were a girl, too."

"At least he ain't drooling on himself anymore. I was noticing now that his face only gets spaced out when he's tired. He has gotten a lot better. Hey, how's he gonna pay his way now that he's canned? I don't think he's gonna have an easy time getting a job."

"Well, you know that house that him and his brother were living in? You know that's the house they grew up in, don't you."

Jeff nodded. "Uh-huh. His dad used to be my Little League coach. Hey, didn't Marty's parents separate after they moved out of there?"

"Yeah. Well, Chris moved out, too. Even he got burned out on Marty. So Marty made a deal with his mom to fix it up and sell it. Marty gets to keep half of the profits to help him get going again."

"I heard he traded his motorcycle for a bicycle. Is that true?"

"He's telling everybody that he's using the bicycle for his rehabilitation. He thinks he's too good for us anymore. I don't know why he can't just play sports to get better."

"I guess you almost can't blame him. I know I don't want to play basketball with him anymore. He almost got the whole gym in a fight last weekend. Don't you remember?"

"Well, yeah, but Krieg should have said something. That was his own fault."

"In a way it was ours, we should have told them. Those dudes from Mount Eden are all sitting there fighting for first pick and who do they pick? I tried not to laugh. They thought Krieg was still good. And if you think about it, he still looks the same, you know, if you don't know what happened."

"All they had to do was watch him dribble."

"Well yeah, they should've been watching instead of trying to hustle first pick, but we really should have warned them. I thought he was going to get killed when that big guy was open and he threw it to the guy that was covering him. If we would've said something I know that fight wouldn't have happened. Those guys on his team were just trying to protect him."

"What's the big deal? At least he didn't get hurt."

After six months of full-time work at my old job at ETEC, I was fired in August 1978. Inside, I was devastated. Feeling I had nothing left to lose, I traded the motorcycle I no longer rode for an Albert Eisentraut fifteen-speed custom frame. It was used but in beautiful condition.

I had decided that I would use my new bicycle to rehabilitate myself. On it, my body didn't pound and jar. The wind, as it passed by my face and through my hair, made me feel alive again. And the bike hid my coordination problems. I could pass for a real biker and a normal person on it.

The first few two-mile jaunts on my bike nearly changed my mind about my capacity for self-healing. My numb hands and sore shoulders and back told me to give up. My ankles scuffed the pedal arms as I wheezed and coughed through each revolution. My throat and lungs felt as if they were on fire. This was no fun.

Remembering my therapy sessions, and Don's admonitions, I kept pushing, and I slowly moved beyond the pain. In five very disciplined months, I aimed for higher and higher aerobic thresholds. As I reached each new plateau, I challenged myself to reach upward to the next level. I recorded my distances daily. As they increased, my body grew stronger and stronger, and so did my confidence.

Despite the fact that I still had a hard time concentrating and comprehending, during the weekends I began to go on organized club rides. In the staging areas, the sound of tire pumps in action and the clicking of gears and humming freewheels made me feel proud. On the road, I watched for how and when the other more experienced riders changed their pedaling cadences. I saw how they drank from their water bottles while still pedaling. I made mental notes of when it was appropriate to coast. Following their example, I pointed out the potholes and glass that appeared in our path.

By the end of the summer, I had established a routine for myself. I got up early as if I were going to work, ate breakfast, read the sports page, and pedaled out of town with the rush hour traffic. Along with gloves, ski cap, windbreaker, and wool leggings to guard myself against the chilly autumn air, I also wore old socks over my bike shoes to keep my feet warm. By the time I made it to the climbing of Palomares Canyon fifteen miles away, I had usually stripped down to bike shorts and a T-shirt.

As much as I tried to ride in the more remote areas away from town, from time to time I still encountered people who knew me. One morning, I had just climbed to the crest of Castro Valley Boulevard, where a fast, winding downhill awaited. A blue fender appeared at my side. I looked back. It was some of the weekend cowboys who lived on nearby Palomares Road.

"Get a job, little Krieg," one of them called out.

I tried to smile and look nonchalant as I kept my eyes on the road that I was now beginning to hurtle down.

"Is that your new car?" another laughed.

Three of them sat in the cab along with a set of gun racks while three more sat in the pickup bed. I recognized a few of them from high school. They often had singled me out to prove their masculinity by belittling mine.

"Get closer, Heinsel, we wanna yank him in the back."

The truck forced me closer and closer to the glass-encrusted shoulder. I tried to slow down and stay out of their way. The truck slowed down with me. Suddenly I felt a hand grab my shoulder. I slammed on my brakes and stopped as they kept going.

"C'mon, Heinsel, stop! He got away!" I heard them yell.

The truck slammed on its brakes and began racing toward me in reverse. Breathing heavily, I pedaled to the safety of the opposite side of the wide, untrafficked boulevard.

"Krieg, you're a pussy. You better not ride your bike on our road today," shouted one of them.

I rode a different route that day.

On weekdays, I tried to ride a minimum of thirty miles a day. I used the afternoon hours to work on the house. Scrubbing walls, hauling trash, and painting fences and bedrooms only left me with enough energy at night to try to improve my reading skills.

Besides working my body, I was also busy rebuilding my personality. My new teachers were the authors of the many self-improvement books that I was now studying. They assured me that problems like people laughing at me, or thinking that I was retarded, would not last as long as I kept my goal, being effective with people, in focus. They also told me that the problems I was having could be expected for anyone who is undergoing radical change in their life. That was comforting.

I could not yet read as well as I once had, and my reading was slow and labored. But in the sentences and paragraphs that I had to read over and over again to comprehend, I began to sense the interconnectedness of body and mind. I saw how my health goals and my personality goals were interrelated. If I wanted to be healthier than anyone the way Don, my therapist, had said was possible, I would have to divorce myself from anything that distracted me from attaining my goal. I could now see how the invitations to go to ball games, movies, concerts, and dinner parties, which had stopped coming a while ago, would only have pulled me from my path.

I didn't want to regain 100 percent of my former self. I wanted more than that. And to reach that goal I became fanatical in my training. My bicycle soon became my only companion. My "friends" began to resent her. Only my mother seemed to truly care about me, and soon she was the only one I spoke with on the phone. I would talk with her every day, and her unqualified love and support helped me get by.

Even though my bicycle didn't have a name, she stayed in my room with me while I read my self-improvement books. If I wasn't exploring back roads with her, we were visiting bike shops or looking for more books about ways to improve my mind. I cleaned her every day, all the while thinking positively about what it would be like to be completely healthy.

After a while, the books challenged me to think bigger and aim higher. What was the biggest way that I could prove to myself and others that I had come all the way back?

In one of the stores my bike and I had visited, adjacent to the meager selection of bicycle books was a section filled with travel books. It was while looking through this section that an idea came to me. Maybe the two of us, my bike and I, could visit some of the exotic places they described. Better yet, maybe we could just find another place to start over.

We would explore the United States together! We could sample the available options by riding from one coast to the other. That way, I could hide what was really an escape plan behind a grand-sounding dream.

Almost immediately, the old tapes of my pre-hospital past began to play. *You can't do that. Adventurers do that type of thing, and what makes you think you're an adventurer? What if you don't make it? Your old friends will laugh you right off the planet.* Other questions began to reverberate inside my head. What roads could I possibly ride my bike on to make it across the nation? Where would I sleep? I surely couldn't afford hotels. How about food? And was my body even capable of such a feat?

In order to find the answers, I started studying my self-improvement books even harder. Somewhere among the highlighted and underlined sentences was the inspiration I would need to pull this next miracle off—if I ever got up the nerve to do it. I finally found the words I would need in three different places.

I copied them down on paper in big letters and placed them throughout my house and on my bicycle. The mirror in my bathroom read, *Whatever you can do or dream you can, begin it. Boldness has genius, power, and magic in it.* On the refrigerator, a magnet held up the words, *Do the thing and you will have the power.* And on my handlebars I taped the affirmation, *Do what you're afraid of.*

These words, and the "DO IT NOW" sign which I had already made, would provide the encouragement to help me achieve my dream.

As talk of a transcontinental—or TransAmerican, as I called it—bike ride now replaced the rehabilitation tales that I once bored people with, I began to meet people who wanted to help me realize my dream. Someone told me about a book that a woman wrote about her 1976 bike ride across the U.S. with a touring company called BikeCentennial. I began to consider touring with their group.

Then I met a man named Leslie Eric Bohm at a bike shop. He was selling bike touring bags for a small company he had started called Eclipse Panniers. He assured me that it was possible to ride across the United States, and that I didn't have to do it as part of a group or only on certain roads.

But I was still unsure. I refused to commit myself to a specific departure date. I did, however, begin to prepare for a long bike ride. I increased the length of my rides, and I began to sleep on the floor in my sleeping bag. With my new challenge in mind, I began to ask questions of those bike club riders patient enough to listen to me. They told me that I needed to build my confidence by taking some of the longer club rides that would be coming up in the spring.

Eager to prove my readiness to myself and others, I took on my first hundred-mile ride—a "century." This one was geared toward the hard-core cyclist and lacked food, water, or first aid stations. Unlike most such rides later in the season, the course itself was not marked, and there was no support vehicle to pick up stranded riders. The ride organizers supplied an overview map of the course, along with a list of the roads to turn on.

My confidence began to soar after the first twenty-five miles. Sparked by the enthusiasm of the twenty or so other riders, I felt strong. By the time I hit the fifty-mile mark, however, I had fallen way behind. I had lost sight of all the other cyclists. Alone on the desolate roads outside of Livermore, thirty miles from home, my body began to feel like the drab, gray sky overhead.

When I began the ride, I hadn't understood that the ride officials would locate the containers of food we were to bring at predetermined drop-off points along the way. I hadn't brought any food, and as a result, I was starving. The hunger I felt gave way to lightheadedness, and I headed toward town, where I could get something to eat.

The miles kept accumulating on my odometer. By the time I reached a convenience store, where I filled up on bananas, raisins, peanuts, and candy bars, I had already ridden eighty miles, my most ever. I tried to find my way back to the course, but I got lost. Soon it began to rain. I headed home, feeling like a failure.

When I arrived, exhausted, I looked down at my mileage counter. It read 110 miles. But had I even accomplished anything? I wondered. Even though I had ridden more than a hundred miles in one day, I knew I could not prove it. I took a shower and fell into bed, wondering as I fell asleep if such a questionable achievement could stand up against a 3,000-mile coast-to-coast bicycle journey.

A loud pounding woke me.

"Marty! Come out, Marty, damn it, come out," It was my brother Chris. He pounded harder as I sluggishly got out of bed.

"Get up right now, Marty. It's serious." His voice sounded desperate.

My weary legs dragged me to the door. I opened it, and Chris fell into my arms. "Mom's dead. Come on, man. She's dead."

I was still groggy from my nap. What he said refused to register. I tried hard to understand what he had said. I didn't move.

"Jesus, don't you care?" Chris demanded.

"What do you mean, she's dead?"

"I went to go visit her and her stupid boyfriend's there and there's all these lights in front of the place and he says she died. They wouldn't let me go up and see. Come on, Marty, put some clothes on."

The official cause of Mom's death was an aneurysm. But I somehow felt that my head injury had caused her to lose her will to live. I knew it had broken her heart to see the son whose life she had molded change so drastically. Back in the hospital she had encouraged me endlessly, and she had fought to keep them from amputating my leg. Then I had returned to her with the living skills of a nine-year-old.

The fact that Mom was gone forever was a concept that didn't sink in. The significance of losing her was buried even deeper as I came out of my isolation to help Dad make funeral preparations and notify relatives and friends. Even though my own brush with death had shown me that Mom was going to a better place, my family could not understand my lack of emotion.

"I don't think Marty even cares about Mom," I overheard

my sister Nancy telling Kathy at the funeral home.

"He just doesn't care about much anymore, Nancy. You know how he is. It's like there's someone else in his body," Kathy responded.

Both of their faces showed the wear of true grief. They had been crying for hours.

My car wreck had made me feel numb. I did not cry because I did not feel. It was almost as if my body, overloaded by so much physical pain, was now refusing to let any emotional pain keep it from repairing itself. My mind refused to allow my mother's death to sink in fully.

But over the next few weeks and months it did slowly sink in that Mom was gone forever. I missed her more and more each day. Mom had never interfered with me. She had never contested the path I chose, and for that reason I had often felt like she was the only friend I had left in the world. Now, Mom had left me to those who doubted my every thought or action.

Somehow, I would have to cultivate a strength of my own.

Chapter 6

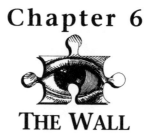

THE WALL

Mom's death made me feel desperate, and it changed the way I looked at things. All of a sudden, nothing mattered to me anymore. I wanted to run away. But where? How? I had talked about riding my bike across the country, but until now that's all it had been, talk. What was holding me back? Had Mom left so that I could become a man and undertake the transcontinental journey I had threatened? I decided to find out. I accelerated my schedule. I'd sold the house in October and moved into a small apartment, and with the money I'd bought a brand-new Honda Accord. A few months after my mother's death I placed an ad in the paper for the car. If it sold, I told myself, then I was supposed to go forward with my ride. It did.

Taking that as my cue, I burned the bridges of retreat, just as my self-improvement books had advised. First, I bought a train ticket north to Portland, where I could begin a more northerly route across America. Then I gave my landlord notice. I gave things away. I sold things. I ignored the warnings from my family and friends that I wasn't ready for a trip across the country. I stopped caring about what people thought. I just forged ahead. By the middle of June I was ready.

The number of material things I had accumulated in my short life amazed me when it became time to put what remained in storage. Dad charged me a high price to safekeep what was left.

"Son, I don't know what the heck's gotten into you. Do you realize that if you change your mind somewhere up there in—where you taking off from, Portland?—that I'm not gonna come and get you?"

Dad fully expected me to turn back partway through the ride I was proposing. He had seen my inability to follow through on anything ever since my car wreck. Armed with a clean slate, and thinking that I had earned a lifetime vacation, in the past few months I had shown Dad a confused young man trying his hand at everything from speed reading and obtaining a real estate license to reentering the master's program and getting back into the accounting field. He had seen me quit every time things got hard.

Dad had grown tired of my talk about becoming a professional bike racer, soccer player, or sports photographer. He saw me make one excuse after another as I tried to explain why people continually fired me. My lack of discipline confused him as he watched me try to figure out who I was and what was important to me in life.

"I can do it, Dad." My speech was still slow, and my enunciation far from perfect. Some people still thought I was slow or retarded when they heard me speak.

"Son, I know you can do it. But what about building a life for yourself? I should have made a plumber out of you. Then you wouldn't have all these problems."

"Yeah, but Dad, after I do this ride I can think about that."

"There's always gonna be something else that you've got to do, Marty. You've got to think about making a living. You're not gonna be able to keep selling things every time you want to take off somewhere. You did that when you got out of college and went to Europe. What the heck kind of life is that, son?"

"This time's different. I have to do this."

"Well, I'll tell ya, Marty, I'm not gonna keep storing things for you every time you want to take off. Build a life for yourself, son. You're past the age for bicycles."

I was crushed. My father's opinion was still important to me.

"Dad, you'll see after I ride across the U.S.," I said as bravely as I could.

"I'll be surprised if you make it even part of the way."

Dad had challenged me. Was he doing it on purpose? He knew that I responded well to criticism.

"And I don't want to be any part of this goof-off little bike ride of yours. You're on your own. I'll store things for you and I want you to call me collect to let me know how you're doing, but that's as far as I'll go."

Inside I knew that Dad was trying to make a man out of me. By telling me in so many words that he could no longer fish me out of tough situations, he was forcing me to grow up. He was trying to make me understand the impact that my actions had on others.

By not offering to support what I was doing beyond an address where I could send and store things, Dad demanded that I think my needs through from start to finish. As my only link to home, he was telling me that I could not count on him to ship me replacement parts if I broke down. And I knew my ride would take me to places where a multi-speed bicycle was uncommon. If I ran out of money, or food, or just got tired of bike riding, I could not call home and ask for a plane ticket.

On June 15 a nearby bike shop put my bike and survival gear into three separate boxes for the train ride north. That's when the problems Dad had forecast began.

"How you getting all these boxes out of here?" Dennis, the owner, asked.

I hesitated. "I... thought I could get a ride from you guys."

He looked at me levelly. "We never talked about that. We agreed to box your bike up for you, but it's up to you to get it out of here."

A lump formed in my throat. I had naively assumed that if a bike shop boxed up one's transportation in this way, then they were also obligated to help that person move around. But that goofy logic didn't seem to make much sense here under the harsh fluorescent lights of the bike shop.

"But... my train leaves in an hour. Now what do I do?"

I had prepared myself for the physical challenge of a long bike ride. Logistical difficulties like these, however, almost proved Dad right. My mind was not yet razor-sharp, and I still made juvenile mental mistakes like this frequently.

"Better get on the phone," one of his mechanics laughed.

"You can use my phone over there behind the counter," Dennis offered.

They had assumed I had friends here. They did not know I was running away. Several unanswered phone calls later, I finally reached Rob, my sister Karen's boyfriend.

"Sure, I'll be glad to help you, Marty, but what about your Dad? Didn't you call him?"

I looked desperately for a good excuse. "I don't think Dad's truck is working."

I felt the bike shop employees listening to me. I didn't tell Rob how I really felt.

"Karen and I will be there as fast as we can make it. You're at Rock's, Alameda, right?"

"Yeah. Thanks, Rob, you're a lifesaver," I said as I hung up the phone.

"You're a wife waver," one of the mechanics mimicked. I often forgot how sloppy my pronunciation was... until someone like that reminded me.

I looked at him. I looked at Dennis, who was also laughing. As I walked outside to wait for Rob, anger at their indifference and cruelty welled up inside of me. I fought the temptation to cry.

"Where you gonna stay when you come back, Marty?" Rob inquired after we'd thrown everything on his truck and taken off.

"Oh. I don't know if I am."

"What do you mean, Marty?" Karen asked.

"I'm sick of this place. I need a change. I'm gonna ride across the U.S. and find the best place to live and hole up there, where people don't know my past and I can start fresh."

When I finished my long, labored speech, Karen began to cry. "What's wrong with us? We didn't do anything to you, Marty," she said between sobs.

"Not you, Karen, not you Rob, just everyone. Dad won't help me, Chris turns all of my friends on me, and Kathy and Nancy, they're always giving me shit about how I don't care about Mom. I got nobody here anymore."

We finished the trip in silence. Soon after we arrived at the train station, a voice over the loudspeaker announced that my train was ready to board.

"Let me help you with some of your stuff, Marty," said Rob. He and I checked my boxes and I turned to say goodbye.

"So will we ever see you again, Marty?" Karen asked. Her eyes were red.

"I don't know," I said, trying not to feel any emotion. I had to follow through with my plan. I had to show those who had brought me love back in the hospital that my life had been worth saving, that I could do bigger things than just get better. I boarded the train and waved goodbye.

As the train slowly lumbered away from the small station, I tried not to let myself think about all that I was leaving behind. I forced myself to look only ahead. The past was over, and I couldn't change any of it.

It wasn't easy. When recollections about Mom, Dad, Chris, Janice, Alex, our dog, my friends, my coworkers at ETEC, or the rest of my family surfaced, I fought them back. Even my death wouldn't have mattered to them, I thought.

As for material things—my car, my apartment, my stereo and waterbed, and the other creature comforts that I had grown accustomed to, I knew they could be replaced.

Even though Dad had coached me on the importance of building a life—which, to me, simply meant hanging onto things—my car wreck had shown me the importance of just letting go. After my life had changed, I realized how little those things mattered when I was faced with the challenge of simply staying alive. Things I had once viewed as necessary now seemed trivial. But other people could not see that.

I slept badly on the train, wrestling with my thoughts all night long. When the train finally made its last stop in Portland, I was ready for something else to occupy my mind. Arrows and signs pointed my way through the throngs of scrambling bodies to the baggage claim area, where I could be reunited with my bike.

"I'm sorry, Mr. Krieg, your third box must have gotten loaded on to the Tacoma train," said the attendant when I showed him that I was still missing a box.

"But that... box has my... wheel in it." I said with an effort.

A look of fear crossed his face as he watched me struggle to produce the needed words.

"Come back tomorrow, it should be here by then. Next!" I was dismissed as some kind of train station drunk.

The panic that began to well up inside me reminded me of my last day at the hospital. Without the right answers then, I knew that I was doomed to more hospital humiliation. And now, even though I knew exactly what I wanted to say, if I didn't speak intelligibly, I would not have a place to sleep or a bike to ride.

I tightened my jaw. I made myself speak more forcefully. "Excuse me," I interrupted as he began to wait on another customer, "I'm riding my bike across the U.S. and I need my front wheel to do it."

That made a difference. I felt proud of myself. The words were loud enough, and he seemed to understand every one of them.

"Sir, in that case you'll have to get that straightened out

with the station manager. His name is Mr. Roth. He handles special cases. Our usual policy is to have you come back tomorrow in the event that something is missing."

"Where?" I asked, using my hospital trick of using as few words as possible and talking with my eyes.

"You can step behind the counter here and follow that hallway. His door is marked."

I thanked him, trying to conceal the pride that I felt in my ability to perform under pressure. I quickly rehearsed what I was going to say next as I walked to the office.

"Come in," a voice called as I knocked on the door. I walked in.

"Hi, Mr. Roth, my name is Martin Krieg and I'm riding across the U.S. on my bike."

I couldn't believe my own ears. I sounded on the outside just like I thought on the inside. That didn't happen often. My efforts, however, had required tremendous concentration.

"Pleased to meet you. How can I help you?" Mr. Roth's burly voice intimidated me. His thick gnarly hands indicated that he had worked his way up through the ranks.

I sucked in my stomach, reminding myself to concentrate.

"You guys loaded my front wheel onto the wrong train and I need it now. I can't wait till tomorrow, I've got to meet some people pretty soon."

I could feel the adrenaline as it pulsed against my forehead. In the pressure of the moment, I had even fabricated a story about why I needed to leave today. Roth nodded as if he understood every word.

Silence overcame the room while Roth pondered my situation.

"I want to help you out, son," he finally answered. "Normally we put out-of-town travelers up in a hotel if their baggage gets misplaced. But I guess I could use that money to buy you a new front wheel if you'd like."

I relaxed. Success! After we negotiated a replacement value, he said, "Well, let's get you going. How 'bout if I drive you to the nearest bike shop?"

My heart skipped a beat. "That would be great."

Knowing that I couldn't call home and ask for help from Dad forced me to perform far above my familiar level of comfort. Successfully negotiating for a replacement wheel showed me that I could win with the countless strangers who would surely be a part of my ride. I decided to use this victory to prepare for the many obstacles that no doubt lay ahead.

As soon as the wheel was put on I took off, even though my heavily laden bicycle did not move smoothly through Portland's rush-hour traffic. I had plenty of supplies with me: my wool cycling cap, shorts, and jersey; leg warmers, socks, gloves, cleats, tennis shoes, undershorts, and T-shirts; a windbreaker, down vest, poncho, and jeans; hand and laundry soap, bathroom kit, sleeping bag, ground tarp, and candles; a small camping stove with kitchen and cooking items; water bottles; a camera and film; my journal; a sewing kit, flashlight, sunglasses, rubber bands, safety pins, Swiss Army knife; and a full bike repair kit that included spare tires and tubes, and patches, lubricants, and tools. For food and emergencies, I carried about eight hundred dollars in traveler's checks. My plan was to try and keep my spending down to ten dollars a day.

It was difficult to maneuver a fully packed touring bike, and it took me a while to get used to it. But before total darkness set in, I was outside the city limits. As the roadside business and traffic lights began to disappear, I found a friendly field and spent my first night on my TransAmerican road in the weeds.

I slept well. At the first light of day I awoke, anxious to get rolling. I still felt sore and cramped from the train ride. I slapped some water on my face and gave my mouth a quick rinse. After I plucked my socks empty of foxtails, I rode northwest up U.S. 30 into the brisk Oregon morning.

Astoria, located at the edge of the Pacific Ocean and in the upper left-hand corner of Oregon, lay about a day beyond the coastal mountain range. That would be my official starting point. BikeCentennial, an organization started in the Bicentennial year of 1976 to promote a healthier lifestyle through biking, started and ended its transcontinental bike rides there. Their route across the continent was cobbled together mostly from older roads with less auto use, and I planned to use some of them on my journey. I had only the vaguest of routes planned: I would bike two days down the coast to Florence, then aim east. I had no plan other that.

After a few miles of sleepy-eyed riding, I reached Scappoose, where I nourished myself and freshened up in a rest room. The riding beyond this small town was glorious. I hooked west over to Highway 47, through the tiny towns of Pittsburg and Mist, to Clatskanie, where I rejoined Highway 30. It was what I'd envisioned transcontinental cycling to be. The vistas were right off a bicycle magazine cover. The warm sun invigorated my tired body, and I savored every tree and fern that made up this rain-soaked private riding sanctuary.

I stopped for a few moments at a bend in the road. Set back from the road, nestled among the trees, was what could have been my dream home. Smoke quietly puffed from the chimney of a small house as a gaggle of ducks sunbathed on its neatly manicured front lawn. In a little pond to the left, I could see water lilies and huge goldfish.

As I rolled away, I began to feel that everything I was doing somehow made sense. I was truly a part of my surroundings. I felt like a participant, not a spectator. Instead of relying on the safety of a picture book or a television set to sharpen my appreciation of the world, I had put all of my senses to work helping me process and appreciate the beauty around me.

My timing for this stretch was perfect, as these ocean-misted gardens were usually blanketed by fog or drenched by rain. The beauty of the countryside, the forest's sweet fragrance, and the absence of cars distracted me from the magnitude of the challenge I had created for myself.

From Clatskanie I followed the Columbia River to Astoria. I made it there in one day, but it was exhausting. I set up camp and got to sleep early, eager for more of the storybook lands I thought lay ahead.

The next morning I headed south on U.S. 101 along the coast, admiring the tranquil ocean views and drinking in the salty air. But after several hours of the noise, wind, traffic, and interminable up-and-down riding, I had second thoughts. I prayed for a change from the breathtaking ocean views that had just that morning stunned me. The cars speeding by kept my eyes pinned to the white line at the edge of the road. Strong head winds and the roller-coaster geography joined in to make my task even harder.

Why had I needed to leave? At least back home, on roads that no longer stimulated me, I had been able to occupy my mind with the exercises that I'd invented to improve the right side of my body. On Palomares Canyon Road, I had forced my face into contorted positions to work my sagging right eye and mouth. On Norris Canyon Road, I would tighten up the right toe strap and pedal with only that leg for miles and miles to rebuild the atrophied muscles in my calf and quadriceps. I worked on my dexterity on Redwood Road by using my right arm to pull my water bottle from its cage. After I guided it to my lips for a small sip, I returned it to its mount on the frame. I practiced this motion over and over again.

But I had neither the time nor the inclination for any of that today. Finally, two hundred demanding coastal miles later and halfway down to California, I straggled into Florence. I spent a night at the state park there, where I slept like a log.

In the morning I turned my bike east. I wasn't on the road long before a great peace overcame me. I was moving away from the coast, and instead of the roaring ocean, I heard bird song. The sun that now warmed my exposed arms and legs replaced the incessant sea winds that had made me feel so exposed.

The open road had also shown me the necessity of a tent. After a couple mornings of waking up in a sleeping bag sopping wet with dew, I decided to invest in my first portable home after I made it to Eugene later that day.

"Do you have any tents I could fit on my bike?" I slowly asked the bespectacled man at an outdoor store there.

His eyebrows raised slightly as he looked at me, then at my loaded bike at the door.

"How long you been traveling?" he asked, scratching his scraggly beard.

"Only about four days and 370 miles. I'm going across the U.S."

"Uh-huh." His response sounded doubtful. "And you've been out for four days without a tent?" He looked at me like I was crazy. I couldn't tell whether he pitied me or wanted me to leave his store.

Because I had not been able to find much information about bike touring, I had been forced to learn as I rode. But I knew he didn't have the patience for an explanation. Did I need to rev myself up for another superhuman effort just so that he could understand me? When would my speech come confidently and easily like everyone else's?

"Do you have any small tents?" I asked, thinking I had found the correct level of effort.

"Of course we do, what do you think backpackers use?

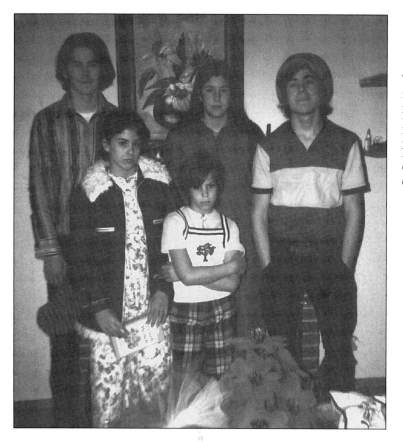

The mid '60s from left, back row: Chris, Kathy, me. Front row: Nancy, Karen. *Credit: Krieg Collection*

Trying to be "a real man" with my van and my motorcycle. *Credit: Krieg Collection*

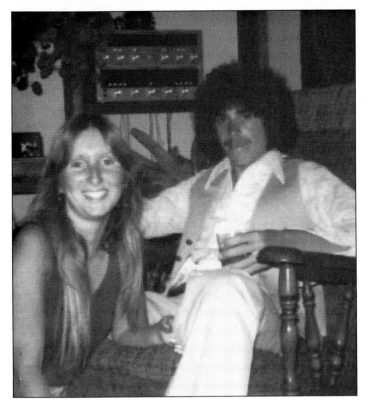

Janice and me
when afros were in.
Credit: Krieg Collection

My best friends
Bob Beaudry and
Jeff Limbeck.
Credit: Krieg Collection

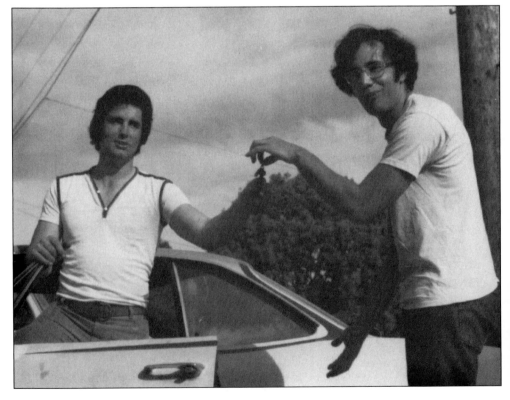

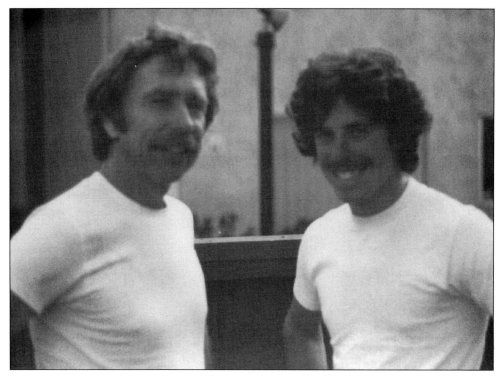

Dad and me on the night before my car wreck. *Credit: Krieg Collection*

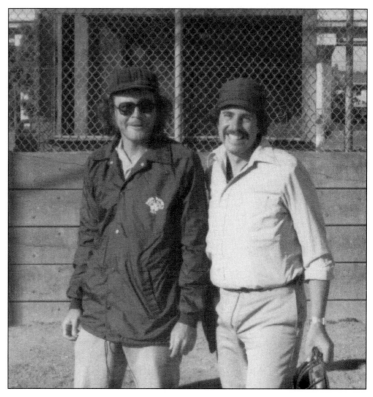

Uncle Jim Jam and
the "rookie"—me.
*Credit: Krieg
Collection*

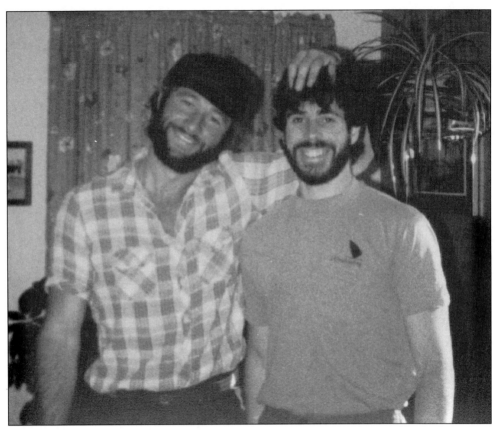

Uncle Dan, aka Gum Chewy/Captain Dan. *Credit: Krieg Collection*

Trailridge in the Rockies with Paul Phillips. *Credit: Krieg Collection*

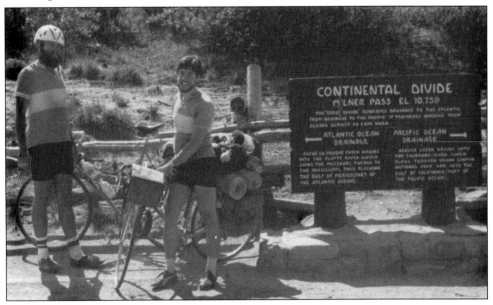

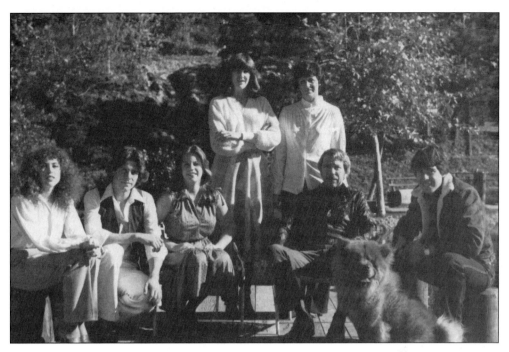

The 1979 Kriegs from left, Nancy, Chris, Karen, Kathy, mom, dad, Alex (the dog) and me.
Credit: Krieg Collection

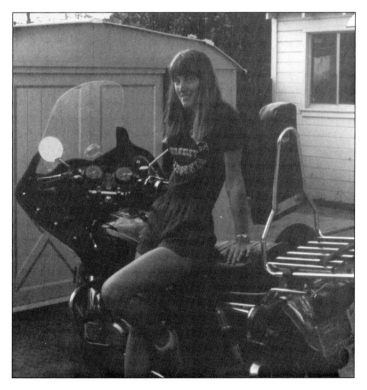

Karen Bauder
on my motorcycle.
Credit: Krieg Collection

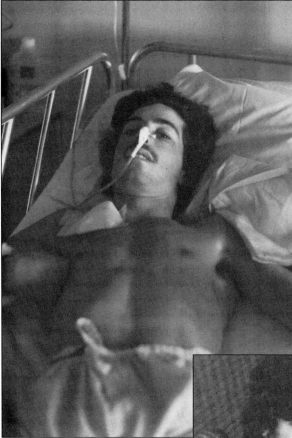

During the coma, my eyes stayed open a lot of the time. *Credit: Krieg Collection*

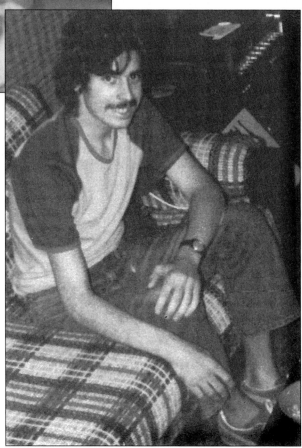

Relaxing at a party given for me, two months after the hospital. *Credit: Krieg Collection*

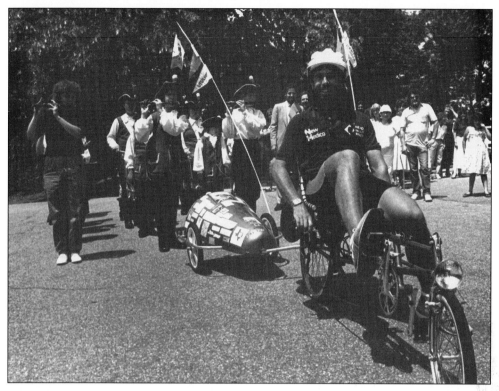

Leading a marching band. Jack Barrette and Peter Gilsey appear just above my right shoulder. *Credit: New Medico Collection*

Meeting Governor Dukakis with Marilyn Spivack, founder of the National Head Injury Foundation, at the State House in Boston. *Credit: New Medico Collection*

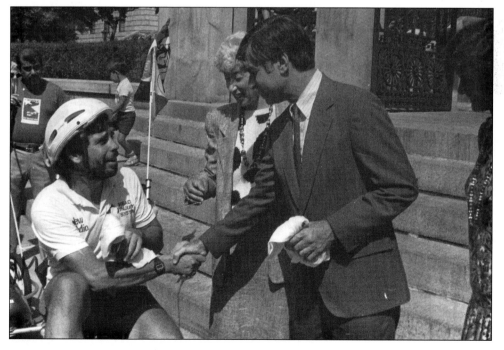

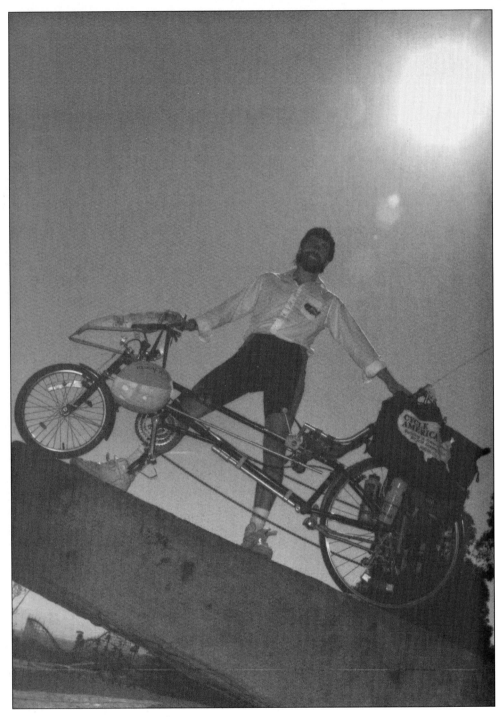

Cycle America, giving the dream of a coast-to-coast bicycle highway a home.
Credit: Todd Tsukushi

That's what this store is all about." He sounded incredulous that I didn't know that.

We soon found a tent that would work. "Is that gonna be it? You better make sure you have everything. That's a mighty long road ahead of you."

"How about maps of Oregon?"

Once again his eyebrows lifted. "You don't have a map of Oregon? How'd you even get to Eugene?"

"I rode the coast. It was easy to figure out. Then I just asked questions."

He studied my eyes as if to see whether I was on drugs.

"If you're gonna ride your bike across the U.S.A., you better start asking lots of questions. It doesn't sound like you're very well-prepared."

A hundred and fifty dollars later, I left his store feeling like a criminal for wanting to bike anywhere without first knowing each and every one of my needs beforehand. I also knew the slow, inarticulate way I spoke had caused trouble for both of us.

I pedaled away from Eugene on U.S. 126 thinking about the significance of my new purchases.

With the tent, I had purchased privacy. My very first home would now help shield me from the campground gawkers who always wanted to know about my bike ride. Since I had so little energy at the end of a day, I could now spread out without having my every personal belonging scrutinized by passersby. Besides the obvious protection that it would give me from the weather, my little yellow shelter would also give me a room in which I could write in my journal at night.

With my maps, I had purchased the freedom to chart my own course. I had naively reasoned that I could just rely on the advice of others for good riding and directions. But the rough coast riding had shown me that there are bike roads and there are car roads and a lot of questions must be asked about each. I was also discovering that the way drivers saw the road was far different from the way I experienced it. They never noticed slight grades that could be murder to a cyclist, and they interpreted distances in minutes, based upon a forty- or sixty-mile-per-hour average speed.

As I studied the maps at night, I began learning how to read the roads ahead. In time, I would know when to expect traffic. A high concentration of towns in an area, no matter how big or small, meant a large volume of cars and trucks. I discovered that roads that curve a lot generally mean up and down climbing because they follow the lay of the land. Federal highways that have been abandoned in favor of interstates, however, usually mean the roadbed has been graded, eliminating steep grades like the ones I had found along the coast. If an interstate closely parallels a major roadway, one can usually expect light traffic.

I always tried to avoid "red" roads. I found that the roads marked in black or blue usually—though not always—represented good riding. The red ones didn't.

Right now, the maps seemed to be telling me that the eastern half of Oregon was made up of desert areas. I was surprised, but I figured anything would be better than the coast. I pedaled on.

I had missed a shower, and the grit of yesterday's windblown ocean sand and the exhaust fumes from today's passing cars covered my pores with a coat of baked-on grime. By midafternoon, my legs felt emptied of any energy by the unrelenting sun.

I wanted to be rested for The Wall, a difficult mountain pass that local cyclists had warned me about, so I began to look for a place to camp.

A few hundred feet after I crossed over the roaring McKenzie River, filled with torrents of white-capped snow melt, a small sign at the edge of the road said "Primitive Campground" and a small trail invited me into a cool forest.

It seemed to promise protection from the blinding sun. Casting aside all caution, I dismounted and followed the trail. It soon ended in a rubble of moss-covered twigs and branches. Off in the distance, I could see light and hear a dull roar. I headed through the dark forest toward the meadow it represented.

The closer I got, the louder the thunder grew. Suddenly, the noisemaker appeared at the edge of the richly carpeted forest floor.

It was the McKenzie, the same river I had just crossed on my bicycle. It had wound its way back to this part of the forest. And the light I'd seen was roaring white water cutting a huge swath right through the middle of the woods.

The trail I had followed had disappeared behind me. I was truly all by myself. I set up my tent right at the river's edge. The despair of having missed a shower gave in to the fear of bathing in the ice melt which roared several feet below. Its unrelenting power intimidated me. My reflexes were still slow, and this was a new and frightening experience. But I knew a cold dip would rejuvenate me. I could not ignore the voice pounding inside my head.

Do what you're afraid of, it said. I gathered my towel and my biodegradable soap and climbed down to the river's edge, where I tested the water with my foot.

Much too cold. I changed my mind. While I'm freezing to death, the raging current will surely sweep me off to an ocean burial, I thought. Besides, no one even knows I'm here. If I get hurt, then what? The reasons I should not take a river bath began to overwhelm me, but that affirmation on my old refrigerator again began to taunt me.

Do what you're afraid of and the fear will be overcome. I knew my fears were only imagined, and I knew a good rinsing would improve my attitude. I looked upriver. Not far off, one of the forest giants had fallen into the river, creating a calm pool to the side. I walked over to see if the water there felt any different.

It didn't. *Do what you're afraid of!* The words screamed in my skull. I took a step back, then surged forward into the river. In a second I was completely submerged.

The cold nearly paralyzed me, and in a frenzy I pulled myself onto the bank using the thick tree roots buried in the sand. The shock had been even more jolting than I'd anticipated, but I immediately began to soap myself down.

Then I stopped. I didn't want to jump back in, but how else was I going to rinse myself? After a few minutes, the sun began to bake the soap in. Before I could think twice I charged even harder into the water and landed farther from the bank. But my brave jump made it difficult to pull myself ashore. My weakened body could barely manage to hold on to the slippery roots. My feet dug even harder into the sandy bottom. I recalled how hard it had been just to scratch my nose back in the hospital, and a sudden burst of energy overcame me. I exploded out of the water.

My body sang out with a new aliveness. My scalp tingled. My hair prickled from it. Every pore in my skin felt alive. My vision seemed to be sharper. The sounds that filled my ears took on an almost concert-hall quality.

Never before had I been so keenly aware of my surroundings. Never before had I so fully understood the power that words had over my life. When I'd done what I was afraid of, the McKenzie River had shown me that I really could challenge, and conquer, my fears. I began to see that the hardest part of any fear was just thinking about it.

I left my campground paradise the next morning rested and eager to take on The Wall. McKenzie Pass climbed 5,324 feet from sea level, and cyclists I had talked to had called it a very challenging ascent. Some had even warned that I would be forced to walk portions of it.

But for now I was still riding mile after mile of a tree-canopied forest wonderland, one that was alive with squirrels and birds. The road switched back and forth as it gently wound through the wooded giants. Moisture from an early shower steamed from the road, and it charged the air with electricity.

Not one car passed me. I had the forest's hypnotic quiet to myself. I was dimly aware that it was the best bike ride of my life, but the fear of The Wall in the back of my mind kept me from fully enjoying it. I kept pedaling.

The sweat gently dripping from my uncovered arms reminded me that this was supposed to be hard. My breathing had fallen into a regular and easy rhythm. It was hard biking, but I kept my speed steady, and I made sure I held a reserve of energy for The Wall.

In the early afternoon, after a morning of constant climbing, the terrain began to change. The steamy gardens and soothing greens gave way to brown clays and jagged rocks. The trees thinned out. My heart beat faster. The Wall must be coming up.

The forest soon disappeared behind me, and I could see that I was nearing the top of the range. I stood up in the pedals, ready for a road grade more difficult than any other, when a summit sign appeared. I slowed down. Where was The Wall? I coasted to a stop at the crest.

I leaned my bike against a huge boulder. The road ahead led down to what looked like a different planet. Off in the distance all I could see were rock formations colored in drab chalky hues. Cracked earth surrounded me, and the glare shining off the flat, massive stones forced my eyes into a squint.

I sat on the dirt trying to make sense out of what had just happened. I had experienced The Wall without even knowing it. One of the best rides I had ever known was over, and I had barely enjoyed it since I'd been filled with dread over what was coming up. I was tempted to turn around and do it all over again, but I reasoned that I would never make it across the country that way.

Had I been guilty of letting others judge what this part of the ride should have been like for me, and therefore what part of my life would be like?

That part of my journey showed me the power, once again, of words. Only this time, it was the words of others. I resolved not to be victimized by them ever again. But I was still unsure of my abilities, and I knew it wouldn't be easy. How could I balance the opinions of others against my own still-developing faculties? That kind of education might take a lifetime. Maybe the miles and trials ahead would bring me closer to the answer.

Chapter 7

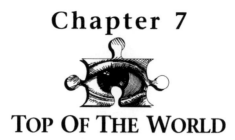

TOP OF THE WORLD

The days and miles of arid desert and harsh glare that followed McKenzie Pass made me long for the green of the forested roads I was leaving. Fortunately, my next destination distracted me from the lifeless surroundings that so exposed me.

I spent a lot of time thinking about St. Alphonsus Hospital and Father Kuiper. Located in Boise, Idaho, just thirty miles over the state line, St. Alphonsus was the hospital that had first ministered to me after my brush with death, and Father Kuiper had said last rites over me while I was there. This small Idaho city, and what it meant to me, seemed to be call out from across the dry nothingness of eastern Oregon.

My daily mileages increased to about one hundred miles as I approached Boise. Every day I felt more oblivious to the heat and barren terrain around me, and I could feel myself getting stronger from one day to the next.

Once I finally crossed the Idaho state line, I bore down on Boise. As it came into sight, I tried to mentally reconstruct my car wreck. I went through each intersection at a snail's pace and studied the shoulders for telltale signs. Maybe I would see a blood stain, a hubcap, a mangled fender. But I saw nothing.

Finally the city limit marker appeared. My heart began to flutter, and my body felt weaker. Dim, unpleasant hospital wheelchair scenes began to replay over and over in my mind.

I couldn't let the people at the hospital see the weakness that I now felt, I thought. I forced myself to draw strength from the successes Don Chu had helped me to achieve. My therapist's words of congratulation and encouragement resounded in my ears. I pulled myself together. By the time I pulled up to the hospital's doors, I felt stronger. I got off my bike and walked it inside.

The receptionist looked up. My soiled clothes, grimy face, and road-stained bike clashed with her antiseptic surroundings.

"Excuse me, sir... we don't allow bicycles in here," she said as I walked closer to her desk.

"Can you tell... Father Kuiper... that Marty Krieg is here," I said, trying to sound as confident as possible.

She paused. My slow, labored speech had caught her off-guard. "Well, all right, but you'll have to do something with your bike."

I nodded at my bike, then looked at her. "This is... my home," I said as she paged the priest.

She looked away from me, only partly masking her disgust. She shook her head and started writing again.

"I used to be a... patient here," I said. Maybe now she'd understand.

"That's good," she said. She didn't bother to look up.

I wanted to tell her that her indifference hurt me. But I knew that I would only make it worse.

"Marty, is that you?" A robust voice called from across the lobby.

The burly, ruddy-faced priest walking toward me hardly looked like a holy man. He was curly-haired and wore glasses, and his thick muscular arms bulged out of his short-sleeved black shirt. If he'd sported a large tattoo it wouldn't have looked out of place.

"Father?"

"You rode your bike here? All the way from California? I don't believe it." He took my hand and shook it vigorously.

"No biggee." I shrugged, then smiled.

"The last time I saw you, we were shipping you back home in an air ambulance. I never did get to hear you talk. You were in a coma. This is incredible! Let's go up to ICU and show off. Look at you," he said, studying my tan skin, road-hardened legs, and bushy beard. For some reason, ever since the accident, the hair all over my body had begun to grow profusely.

"Father, no bikes in the hospital," the receptionist called.

"Have the janitor lock it up in the tool room. Come on, let's go, Marty."

"But... that's my home, I can't leave it just laying around."

"Well, come on then, let's lock it in my office."

After we secured the bike we headed for the elevator. On the way, Father stopped two men in white smocks. "Hey! Don't you remember this guy?"

The confused looks on their faces made it clear they did not.

"This is Marty Krieg."

Still no reaction.

"Come on, you guys. The guy we shipped out of here on an air ambulance last year."

"Oh, I remember the air ambulance. I'm sorry—what was your name again?" One of them reached his hand out to shake mine.

"I'm just Marty," I said. I felt defeated inside. Was I just another job for the people here? I had thought that everyone would remember me.

As we walked away, I tried not to let Father notice my hurt feelings. A part of me wanted to blame him. I felt as if he had just set me up for that one.

"Nancy... Nancy!" he called to a blonde-haired nurse as we stepped off the elevator onto the third floor. She turned as we caught up to her.

"Father, I'm running late, what is it?"

"Don't you remember this guy?"

She shook her head.

"This is Marty, remember Chris from the Bay Area's brother?"

"Sure, I remember Chris, the good-looking guy, right? He was in here every day, wasn't that the deal where he and his brother got in a... ." Her face turned red. "I'm sorry. Marty, right? Well I gotta go. Looks like you're doing pretty good." She turned and looked at Father Kuiper for a second more than necessary. "Well, gotta go, 'bye, Marty." She darted off.

No one remembered me. Did they even care? My face grew hotter as we continued walking down the long, tiled hallway.

"That's where you were at, Marty." Father pointed to a room full of complicated-looking medical machines and a few patients. "Want to go take a look?"

I nodded. I knew I would choke if I tried to say anything.

We walked in. Father said, "You were in that bed there. Turn around. You see that man right there?"

The patient he pointed at looked like he was fighting for each breath. His breathing sounded rough and irregular.

"Things didn't look so good for you either, Marty. That's what you looked like when we first got you in here. You were struggling for each breath. Your mom was right there with you, too."

I looked inquisitively at Father.

"Yeah, she and your father flew right up here. I'll tell you, boy, she was coaching you through each breath. She was saying, 'Come on Marty, breathe, breathe.'" He paused. "And yes, I heard... Chris called me with the bad news. Your mother was a wonderful lady."

Father Kuiper and my family had gotten pretty close while I was in here. He had gotten to know them better than he had me. I ached inside.

"Father, let's go," I managed to say. I got my bike and left as soon as I could. Father Kuiper waved as I pedaled away.

Instead of letting St. Alphonsus continue to devastate me, I ground the pain up in the rugged Sawtooth Mountains west of Boise. Over the many miles of demanding riding ahead, my thoughts drifted to my hospital visit over and over again. Had it shown me that I was not the center of the universe, that life really did go on without me? And if that were so, how could I make others feel that it was important that my life had been saved?

There was little of nature's beauty to soothe me. The sparse forest grew out of a red rock carpet that hardly looked inviting. It was early July, and the sun beat down mercilessly. The day after Boise I began to dream about the Lowman hot springs. A couple of cyclists back in the Portland area had rapturously extolled the life-giving properties of these natural hot baths. They would soothe my every ache, they said.

My mind's eye saw a scantily clad Greek goddess feeding me grapes while another massaged my worn-out legs. Water gushed out of a hillside and flowed between rocks of gold and silver. An icy pool next to a giant shade tree allowed me to alternate the hot with the cold, speeding my rejuvenation. A pure mountain spring ran down one of the granite walls. Its crystal-clear liquid tasted like golden honey.

I was jarred out of my reverie by the sight of another cyclist ahead. He was standing into each revolution of the pedals. A massive, overstuffed pack sat on his back. I tensed myself against the pedals and rode harder to overtake the bizarre-looking rider. I soon caught him.

"Where you headed on that thing?" I huffed as I drew abreast.

"Oh, I'm just getting out of the Air Force and I'm headed back to Michigan," he answered.

His name was Bryan. I looked at his department store bike. I wondered how he had made it this far. It looked like all the possessions of his military life were in, on, and around his huge backpack—thick-soled military boots, a generous assortment of cast-iron pots and pans, and miscellaneous jackets and sweaters and pants hung from or out of his pack. Several large, heavy metal canteens clanked against the pack's metal frame.

The weight nearly knocked him over when we stopped.

"Bryan, you gotta ship some of that stuff back home. What's that weigh, four hundred pounds?"

He laughed. "I don't know, but it's heavy." He staggered off the bike and struggled to get the pack off his back. "But I can't afford a car and I got all summer, so what the heck."

"Can't you send that stuff home?"

"Well, my mom moved and I don't have her new address."

"When you get into the next town, put that stuff in boxes. Find the post office and send it to your hometown via general delivery. You can address it to yourself. That way, you can pick it up when you get back home." I paused, realizing how knowledgeable I sounded. I even got all the words right. "But the post office in Lowman is going to be closed for July Fourth, and my maps show nothing but hills until Galena."

"I'll just keep going till I find one that's open then. I'm in no hurry. If I get too tired I'll just sit down. If I just keep plugging along, I know I'll make it. But thanks for the tip. I didn't know about general delivery."

Bryan's wiry body looked like it was on overload. His glasses and short hair gave him the look of a librarian. He was shorter than me, maybe 5'4". I knew pure desire had driven him to this point.

"Are you headed for the hot baths right now, though?" I asked.

"Hot baths?"

"You haven't heard of the Lowman hot baths?"

He shook his head. "No, what's that?"

"Man, they come right out of the ground. These guys back in Oregon told me that they'll take the kinks out of your legs and everything."

Whenever I met up with other cyclists on the road, the conversation always progressed at a furious pace. It seemed that both parties wanted to expend the least amount of time in determining the road and people conditions ahead. Somehow I always managed to overcome my speech problems in such instances. During the long rides between such exchanges, I often wondered how I could properly shape my vowels and consonants when the pressure was not on me. Maybe I could pretend that each person I had dealings with was a road-wise bicycle traveler.

"Sounds like just what I need. How far are they?"

I gave him directions. We agreed to meet there after I pedaled ahead on Highway 21 and got us a camping spot.

As I neared the tiny one-store town of Lowman, I asked several people where the fabled hot baths were. No one knew what I was talking about. They looked at me in a familiar way—like I was crazy or retarded. But they did say that the state park, located just up the road, had some small warm pools that I might be able to soak my feet in. I remained optimistic as I pedaled off to the state park.

I coasted over a small bridge into the park and rested my bike against a picnic table several yards off the trail. Just then a group of black-leather-jacketed motorcycle riders rumbled across the bridge. They gunned their engines as they roared past. I remembered how I, too, used to scare people with my power bikes, and I wore my best tough-guy smile.

Since I now had company I didn't trust, I decided to wait until Bryan arrived before I went off in search for the hot baths. An hour passed. Then two. The longer I waited, the more committed I was to staying the night here. Fifty miles and another mountain pass separated me from the next available camping, and I was running out of daylight.

Nearly four hours after we had left each other, Bryan's hulking figure rounded a corner on the road below.

"Bryan," I shouted. "Up here."

Even though he was standing into the pedals on the gentle road grade below, his pace remained slow. I agonized through each revolution. Finally, he made it into the park. He sluggishly made his way toward our campsite.

"Looks like we got company," Bryan said as he looked at the motorcycle party getting into full swing fifty yards away.

"Yeah... I didn't go look at the hot baths yet. I had to keep an eye on things. What took you so long?"

"I told you, I'm not fast, but if I say I'm gonna be

somewhere you can count on it. I just keep plugging."

"I was wondering how you were going to make it over all those passes. Good job, guy. Hey, I'm dying to check out those hot baths. I'll be back in a bit."

At the edge of the creek, I found the small hot pools that the locals had talked about. They were small, all right—they weren't even deep enough for my feet. I walked back up to the main part of the park and asked the first person I saw about hot baths. Same answer. Small hot pools, no hot baths that he knew of.

I asked the motorcycle group. They laughed at me like I was crazy.

"Ain't no hot baths anywhere around here. You better ride your bicycle back down to Boise and get a hotel if you want hot water," one of them cracked. The rest laughed wickedly.

"I used to ride motors, you guys." I tried to sound tough. "But I knew I was gonna go down if I kept riding 'em, so I quit. I'm riding across the U.S. right now."

Even though I had slurred my words, they were already too drunk to care.

"I went across Idaho and back in one day," a short balding man with a huge stomach said as he stepped to the front of the group.

"On a bicycle?" I tried to sound impressed.

"No, man, I don't ride no fairy bikes, I did it on a Harley." He looked back at his buddies and smirked. The group burst into laughter again.

"I'm riding a bike because I'm trying to get better from a head injury. I got all messed up." I tried to take a different approach. Maybe if I got them to feel some compassion for me, Bryan and I would be able to sleep peacefully tonight.

"Ain't that what Georgie got, a head injury?" the fat man asked the group. Turning back toward me, he growled, "Yeah, and Georgie's still in the hospital. That guy used to be a party animal. You and your buddy camping here tonight?'

"I think so."

"All right, we'll leave ya alone. Out of respect for Georgie," he said, "but we still don't like your little fairy bikes, right guys?"

"Fuck fairy bikes," another said. More laughter.

I gave up on the hot baths.

We quietly set up camp, ate our dinner, and retired to

our tents. As soon as nightfall approached, motorcycle thunder rumbled past our tents, startling me from my sleep. I peeked out my little fabric door and saw that the original seven bikers were now almost twenty. I put my head back on my pillow, wondering what to do next. I said a prayer, then another. Finally, exhausted from a week of hard riding, I fell back to sleep.

Somehow, I slept soundly.

When I awoke the following morning, I peeked outside to survey the damages. Strewn about were empty beer bottles and burned, shredded paper from countless fireworks remnants. How had I slept through fireworks? There were still twelve motorcycles left, and next to each was a passed-out rider. Some protected themselves from the dew with a sleeping bag, others lay motionless in their leather biker outfits.

"Bryan... you awake?" I whispered in the direction of Bryan's tent.

"Yeah... are our bikes still there?"

"Uh-huh... let's get out of here, they're all asleep."

Bryan quietly clambered out of his tent and walked over. "It looks like hell out here. Let's go. How fast can you break your tent down?"

"Wait and see. Let's just not wake 'em up and let's get going."

I climbed out of my tent and checked the air in my tires. No problem. Bryan checked his. No problem.

I silently thanked Georgie, their head-injured friend.

A short while later, after we had packed our campsites back onto our bikes, we silently and swiftly pedaled out of the park. Once we were safely out of earshot of the bikers, Bryan and I stopped and laughed about our night.

"I never thought we were going to make it," Bryan said. "I just kept hearing this guy saying, 'No, leave those fairy bikes alone.' What did you tell them?"

"I told 'em about my head injury and they said they wouldn't bother us because they got a friend who has one."

"Weren't you shitting bricks, though?"

"I guess I slept through it all."

"Man, you should have heard 'em. Sounded like Vietnam out there. They were doing firecrackers and bottle rockets. I heard their bottles landing down there in the creek. There was this one guy, I didn't dare look out of my tent, he kept racing his motorcycle to the end of the park and skidding. I can't believe you didn't hear them. I can't even believe we're still alive."

We talked about Bryan's sleepless night for a while before we decided to part company.

"Well, I don't want to hold you back. Where you headed now?" Bryan asked.

"Looks like Idaho has a desert and I've got to go through it if I want to make it to Yellowstone." I pronounced the park's name like Elmer Fudd would have, and we both laughed. "I've never seen it before, so that's where I'm headed now."

By now Bryan was my friend. Since he knew about my head injury, he understood why, at times, some words didn't come out quite as planned.

"Well, let's stay in touch. And as soon as I get to a town I'll send some stuff home," he said.

"General delivery. Well, thanks for the company out here. I'll write. Good luck." I shook Bryan's hand.

I spent the rest of the day climbing into the center of the Sawtooth Mountain range. I thought about Bryan, and what he had shown me about the importance of a man's desire. He had shown me that his will was bigger than his machine—and his backpack. Gauging my efforts against Bryan's, it embarrassed me to think that, with my custom, fifteen-speed touring machine, I was not already halfway across the United States.

As I shifted into my lowest gear to tackle the rest of 7,000-foot-high Banner Summit, a different set of questions occurred to me. The Lowman baths had been very disappointing. Had I looked toward the future at the expense of the present? Was it wrong for me to think that it was always going to be better just a little ways down the road? Why couldn't I have figured out a way to just enjoy the rock-carpeted roads that had led up to Lowman?

What was I running from, anyway? Where was I running to? Did I even know what I was looking for? A line from *The Wizard of Oz* came to mind: *If you're looking for your heart's desire, don't look any farther than your own backyard.*

But I still had a lot of other lessons to learn. I pressed on.

After an afternoon of steady climbing in the hot Idaho sun, my water bottles began to run dry. The next town, Galena, was about forty miles away. Only the emergency quart strapped onto my sleeping bag kept me from panicking.

As I gazed at the distant, snow-covered peaks that I would have to mount, something wet sprayed the backs of my legs. I looked down at my pedals and noticed that they were soaked. I stopped, and climbed off my bike. The plastic water bottle that I was counting on had slipped onto the rear tire and burst open.

A chill ran down my spine. My breath became irregular. I could feel myself panicking. Then I remembered how, back in the hospital, I couldn't even let people know I was thirsty.

It dawned on me that something would work out, just as it had then. Maybe an automobile would come along and I could get them to help me. Maybe a spring would appear on the side of the road. I climbed back on my bike and began to pedal.

About a mile up ahead I saw a car pull out of a clearing on the side of the road. Another one joined it. I focused on this vortex of activity.

As I grew nearer to the clearing, both cars disappeared into the distance. I remained hopeful. Maybe there was a house up there where I could get some water.

A few minutes later I reached the mystery spot. All that remained was a large, red pump. There was no house. The small slab of concrete on which this mechanism sat appeared wet. It looked out of place.

If there really was water in there, surely it couldn't be drinkable. Maybe those cars had used it to fill up their radiators. Maybe the forest service just used it to fight fires.

I dismounted and walked over to the pump. I worked the large red lever up and down. A powerful gust of ice water exploded out of the nozzle and sprayed my legs and feet. Seconds later, a car magically pulled into the clearing.

"Hey... do you know if this water is any good?" Maybe these folks could help me out of my plight.

A man climbed out of the beat-up station wagon. "You won't find better water than this anywhere, son. I come here to fill up my jugs every week. I been drinking this stuff for years."

He looked healthy and fit. He was probably in his fifties. His voice was forceful, and he had a full head of hair. The water didn't look like it had hurt him.

"All right." I went back to my bike to fetch my four small water bottles.

"I won't take long, I just have these little water bottles to fill up," I said as I held the first one under the pump nozzle. The water was so cold that icy beads of condensation collected on the outside of the bottles. I took a gulp and instantly understood what he had meant.

The frosty water tasted pure, just the way nature had designed it. It coated the passage from my mouth to my stomach with a soothing, nectar-like sweetness. Was it possible ordinary water could taste this good? The taste buds in my mouth felt like they had been awakened from a long sleep.

I looked at the man. "This stuff is incredible!"

He nodded. "Yup. It tastes the best right here at the pump. You let it sit around in a container and it seems to lose some of its fire. I usually stay here for a while and celebrate the simplicity of water like this, like it's meant to be. Makes you really appreciate the things that we all take so much for granted, I'll tell ya."

"I don't want to leave, either. Do you mind if I stick my head under it for a second?"

"Be my guest."

The water that gushed over my head reminded me of the McKenzie River ice bath I had taken a week ago back in Oregon. Once again, my scalp tingled with aliveness. The water that coated my face seemed to pull every nerve fiber to the outermost bounds of my skin.

I left this mystery water pump feeling recharged and alive again.

Water took on a new meaning for me. I could remember how, in the past, I had always preferred a soda or a beer to a glass of nature's very own special reserve. I had thought that since water was free, it was unimportant. I was beginning to understand that water was the foundation of everything, that it was the very basis of life. Like the gratitude I now felt for being able to hold a full drinking cup up to my mouth, I felt appreciation for a most basic need: Water.

Along U.S. 93, between the wide-open grassy plains of the Stanley Basin and the snow-capped peaks overlooking Sun Valley, I descended into more desert. Again I imagined luxurious oases ahead. A half-day's ride would bring me to Craters of the Moon National Monument. I envisioned willow trees, sprawling lawns, and tranquil ponds. Wrong.

There was only a small visitors center and a dust bowl for a campground. I filled up on water and pedaled off to the desert town of Arco, fifteen miles away, where I spent the night.

The desolate road that led east from Arco, Highway 88, greeted me with this sign: "NOW ENTERING U.S. DEPARTMENT OF ENERGY TESTING LABORATORY". Idaho had condemned this part of their state to nuclear testing. An eerie feeling settled over me as I passed unnamed roads that veered off to countless empty Ground Zeros. For a day I worried about radiation levels, then returned to the land of the living in Rexburg, thirty miles from the Wyoming border.

Soon the Tetons appeared on the horizon. They grew larger as I pedaled toward them. When I then turned and headed north toward the Montana entrance to Yellowstone National Park, they formed a powerful backdrop to the irrigated fields on either side of me. Finally climbing through them, the thing that made the Tetons hard for me was the unending procession of cars and trucks, many towing boats and trailer homes. Like those on the Oregon coast, they forced me to keep my eyes glued on the white line at the edge of the road.

Because the road had no shoulder, I distracted myself from the boredom with sunflower seeds. I filled my mouth with them whenever there was a break in the action. Using my tongue, I maneuvered, cracked, chewed, and swallowed one after the other as I pumped away. Listening to the struggling of engines on the steep grade was satisfying, and it motivated me to push even harder to demonstrate the superiority of my mode of transportation.

I was almost at the top when a hostile welcoming committee of large horseflies began to bite and bother me. I should have heeded their warnings. What I could see of the park was disappointing. I ventured no further than its main roads, and found nothing there but traffic and crowds.

I anxiously headed directly south on Highway 89 toward Utah. On the wide-open roads out of Yellowstone, I thought about the exchanges I'd had there. The disturbed look on a storekeeper's face when I asked him a question... the driver who stopped me to ask directions and laughed at my slow answer—what could I have done differently? I replayed similar scenes back home with family and friends to try to come up with a more effective outcome. The more I thought about my problems with people, the more I could see that I caused them. What, then, was I running from? Somewhere I had read that our separateness is only an illusion anyway, that we all come from the same place... if that was so, what was the point? My thoughts began to wander in circles.

It was in Jackson, just south of Grand Teton National Park, that I finally found a good bike shop. I'd been looking for one for more than a week. I had failed to bring a chamois to absorb sweat, and my riding shorts had rubbed my butt raw. Since Oregon, I'd had a bleeding rash. My body was almost always in pain—there was a constant throb in my ankle, a dull, steady ache in my shoulders, and a fire along my spine—but my "diaper rash" had been the worst. The chamois made the rest of the ride bearable.

A few days later, after I'd dipped down into the northwest corner of Utah on Highway 44 into the heat-blasted rocks of Vernal, I turned east for good. I crossed into northern Colorado at Dinosaur on U.S. 40, then made Craig the next day. That's when I began to psych myself up for the biggest challenge of the trip—the Rocky Mountains. For the two days that preceded them, I thought of nothing else. I knew that if I made it over them without stopping to walk, I could view my physical rehabilitation as complete. It was something I wanted desperately.

From Steamboat Springs I continued on 40 and ascended Rabbit Ears Pass, 9,550 feet, amid breathtaking views of richly forested mountain valleys. While their earthy fragrance saturated my lungs, I had not once been tempted to walk. The Rockies—at least this first leg—seemed no more difficult than the Sawtooth or Tetons before. Victory seemed probable.

At a store in the small mountain crossroads town of Kremmling, on the Muddy River, I met Paul.

"Where you headed?" the large man asked. He dwarfed the bike he straddled.

"I'm pedaling across the U.S... Now I'm trying to figure out the best way to get through the Rockies," I answered.

I looked at his bike. His huge hands gripped the handlebars of a bike made for heavy-duty use. The spoke count in his wheels looked double the normal amount. The thick braking mechanisms looked like they could stop a five-ton truck. The frame's head tube looked as long as my forearm, while the bike itself towered over me.

"I'm doing Trailridge tomorrow, that's the highest highway in the world," he said in a deep, throaty voice. He looked like one of the giant people I had seen in the wax museum in San Francisco.

"I thought Banner was the highest," I said knowledgeably.

"Oh, I already climbed that. No big deal. I've been out here climbing all these mountain passes, that's how I spend my vacation every year. I come out here and ride the Rockies. And of all of 'em, Trailridge is the toughest." He scratched his thick, curly beard.

I wondered if he was baiting me. Then I heard those familiar words: *Do what you're afraid of, and the fear will be overcome.* But why press my luck? I only needed to prove to myself that I could get through the Rockies. That would be enough; anything else would be actively searching for a way to fail.

"Want some company?" I heard myself say.

Paul looked at me, and a smile crossed his face. "Think you can handle it? It's a big pass and the higher you get, the harder it gets to breathe. I don't know… " He shook his head.

"Paul, I just got done being paralyzed and in a coma for two months. I think I can do Trailridge," I said, using my old standby of selling myself with my car wreck. I told him about my rehabilitation.

Then he looked at me and said, "If you can do what you did, let's do Trailridge."

Paul orchestrated the drama for my ensuing challenge perfectly. Before we camped at the Grand Lake campgrounds, located at the base of the pass, Paul said, "Let's stop in Granby and pick up some fresh vegetables for stew tonight. We're gonna need a solid meal in our stomachs for tomorrow's climb."

I could see that the mountain-sized man took this pass seriously.

At the campground, as Paul cut our huge bagful of corn, squash, carrots, and onions into camp stove-sized chunks with his Swiss army knife, he said, "You better go over every nut and bolt on your bike. You can't afford to have any failures up there."

As he said that, one of his small saucers fell onto the ground.

"Damn. I wanted that for tomorrow's oatmeal." He fished

it out of the pine needles. "We're gonna be leaving pretty early tomorrow, and I'm trying to have as much stuff done as I can before we leave. It'll be so cold then that you won't even be able to feel your hands. I suggest you set your clothes all out ahead of time. You might even pack yourself a lunch that you can munch on from your handlebar pack. We'll be riding the pass for most of the morning."

"What do you mean, cold?"

"Altitude. We're already up at about 10,000 feet. It gets really cold at this altitude, no matter what the season is. Don't you remember? But wait'll you see Trailridge. It climbs over two miles above sea level, and I'll tell you, it looks like the Arctic tundras up there. Even though it cuts through Rocky Mountain National Park, they have to close it most of the time because they have these wild storms up there."

Peeling oranges and bagging up my sandwiches and raisins as Paul had suggested, I prepared the food that would fuel me over the top. Then we ate Paul's stew. It was the best meal I'd had in a long time.

"I can't believe you did this on a camp stove," I said slowly. "I don't cook this good at home."

Paul grinned. "When I've got to come up with something to get me over a mountain, I always come through."

I fell asleep that night feeling fortunate for the opportunity to take on the greatest test of my physical rehabilitation with a road pro like Paul.

I awoke several times during the night, wondering if it was time to get up. Finally, at the first hint of daybreak, I climbed out of my tent into the frozen morning. Paul was already up.

"Start dressing in layers," he said solemnly. "As the climb warms you, you'll want to start stripping down."

"You were right last night. I can hardly feel my hands." I rolled up my tent and sleeping bag.

Paul started a small fire, then cooked up a small pot of oatmeal. It warmed up my insides.

"Let's do it," Paul said as we finished clearing out our campsite. The time for my supreme test had come.

"Shouldn't we wait until it warms up a little?" I was getting cold feet, and it wasn't just from the altitude.

"You'll warm up just pedaling. Besides, if we wait, it'll be nothing but cars up there. Come on, let's go."

"How 'bout if I meet you?"

"Suit yourself, but you're just gonna get colder."

Why was I stalling? Was I afraid to see myself fail? How could this mountain inflict any greater pain on me than I had already endured?

"You're the expert. Let's go." A minute later we were off.

For the first few miles, the road climbed gently. Not too bad, I thought, I could do this. I tried not to get excited. I paced myself. I kept my thoughts focused on one thing— the road just ahead of me. I didn't stop at the observation points along the way; I was afraid that the cars there would upset my momentum. As I slowly pedaled by, I could hear people complain about the breathing difficulties the altitude caused. Some of them offered words of encouragement to us. Others who just stared in disbelief made me feel stronger.

Once I climbed above tree level along the winding road, I knew nothing could stop me. The jubilation that began to well up inside of me, however, was tempered by the otherworldly tundra all around. My thoughts wandered as I approached the top.

I remembered how my lack of wind had made it difficult for me to speak in sentences or walk up a flight of stairs. Here I was, powering that same body over the highest highway in the world. I was even beating a man the size of the mountain itself.

Paul's weight was slowing him down. He was toiling away several turns below me.

At the ranger station near the top, I could see that there was little of the mountain left to climb. My heart began to pound. I had made it. I felt a tremendous urge to share my achievement, and I stopped at the little rock building to join the handful of other cyclists whose bikes I saw parked outside. They had conquered Trailridge from the other side.

I decided to wait there for Paul. Inside the small building, I could sense the pride that each cyclist felt.

"All right, Paul," I said as he walked inside ten minutes later. His breathing was labored, but he smiled at me.

"Marty, you did it. Congratulations." That was all he could get out for a while.

I heard one cyclist ask another how long he'd been on the mountain. Inside, each of us compared the answer to our own experience. For me, my triumph was not about time. Trailridge had shown me that my physical rehabilitation was complete. When I'd started off weeks ago I'd been relatively weak and unconditioned. But the daily hours of long, hard work had whipped me into shape. For the first time I felt like I was on even footing with people whom I had once viewed as superior just because they could walk. The confidence I had gained from the physical challenges of biking these western U.S. would help me deal with the more densely populated areas ahead.

It was the best I'd felt since my early rehabilitation triumphs. I celebrated on the long downhill that took me off the mountaintop, speeding along as fast as I'd ever traveled on a bike. I felt invincible. I shot my fist into the air and shouted words of celebration as I rode down the mountainside in triumph. I took my hands off the handlebars and careened downhill with my hands in the air like a racer completing his victory lap. At that moment I felt that I could do anything.

Chapter 8

CLOSE ENCOUNTERS

The Midwest added an element of predictability to my riding. Since many of the smaller towns were marked by a towering silo or a grain elevator, I knew far in advance where I could fill up on water. The vast oceans of soybeans and corn that surrounded these farm belt skyscrapers seemed to have provided well for the farmers of Nebraska and Iowa. Many of their towns were marked by a swimming pool complex complete with sprawling lawns and picnic tables. I almost always ended a day of riding at one.

It was at these parks that I began to experiment with some of the people skills I was learning. Before I could graduate to people my own age, I practiced on children. I found that if I took an interest in them and looked only for the good, they would reciprocate and overlook my deficiencies.

I was a favorite with them at most campgrounds. They would wash my dishes and empty my trash and listen spellbound as I told them of my adventures. Their attention rebuilt my confidence. My self-esteem soared even higher every time I awakened to a note of encouragement from one of their parents or a care package or an address with an invitation to write. When people my own age invited me for dinner, I usually made up an excuse. I still was not ready, and dealt with adults only when it was unavoidable.

After more than a week's trekking across the Central Plains, I crossed the Mississippi River at Keokuk, in the southeastern corner of Iowa. There, the city parks disappeared. I had to rely on the farmhouses of Illinois, Indiana, and southern Ohio to get me across the rest of America's Breadbasket.

The first Illinois farmhouse that I stopped at showed me what kind of response I could expect.

I was trying to keep up with a tailwind as I headed away from the Mississippi River. The sight of a water pump near Lincoln stopped me. It stood in front of a farmhouse along a deserted stretch of Highway 10. I was dried out by the wind, and I hoped it would deliver the same kind of liquid rush that the pump in the Stanley Basin had.

I leaned my bicycle along the hedge that marked the property line. As I walked up to the white clapboard cottage, a tidy, attractive woman with a teacup figure came outside to greet me.

"I was wondering if I could fill up my water bottles from your pump over there. I'm going across the U.S. and I'm from California," I said. I'd found that delivering my credentials almost always helped.

Inside I thanked the kids from the Corn Belt states who had helped me practice my speech without undue pressure. I had a ways to go, but at least people didn't look at me as if I were retarded and look around for the closest escape route. The woman didn't even blink before she answered my question.

"Please, be my guest," she said. "After you help yourself to all the water you want, why don't you stay and chat for a bit? We don't see many long-distance travelers out here and I want you to meet my husband. He's awfully proud of that little pump. And I don't think that he's met a bicyclist from California before, either."

"Are you sure? I'd love to stay a little, but I gotta keep on moving if I'm gonna find a good place to camp. When does your husband come home?"

"Dale will be here any minute. We can all have dinner together. You can camp here under our willow tree, if you like. Oh, do stay." She smiled brightly.

As we waited for Dale, I told the woman about my rehabilitation and all of the successes I was having with this ride.

When Dale finally came home, he looked at me like he wasn't sure what his wife, Georgia, had gotten him into. A tall, handsome man with square, work-hardened shoulders, he barely said hello. They excused themselves.

While they were gone, I decided that winning Dale over would be my challenge this evening. Building on my successes with all the kids back in Nebraska and Iowa, I knew what I would do. I would ignore all the negative messages that he was giving me and focus only on the positive. I would find out what he liked to talk about. I would learn about him.

When they returned, Dale seemed even more hostile.

"Don't you work?" he said. His eyes shifted over towards the garage, where some more chores awaited him.

"I used to be an accountant, and now I'm just trying to get myself back together so I can start working again." I smiled at him. "Georgia tells me that you own a lawnmower shop over in Champaign. How long have you owned that?"

"About five years. Which reminds me, I've got to get a motor out of my trunk."

"Need some help?"

"No, I can handle it."

I walked outside with him anyway. "Georgia tells me that you used to be a schoolteacher like her and that you just said to hell with all the politics."

"That's right," he said as he walked toward his car.

I followed him. "That's kind of what I'm doing. I got sick of counting someone else's money for 'em and I want to get back into something where you really work with your hands or something when I get back."

He studied me as he fumbled with the tie-down ropes.

"I think I'll take you up on your offer. Why don't you grab this side, this thing is a lot bigger than I remembered. This is sure a lot easier than that hoist there," he said as we lifted the small engine into the back of a wheelbarrow.

That seemed to warm him up. Soon he was asking me questions. I knew I had won his friendship when he volunteered to drive me into town to get some parts for my bike.

"Thanks, Dale, but I can't take rides from cars, that's against the rules."

"Is that so? Well, if you break down out there and need a lift, you know where to find us, State Highway Ten," Dale joked as he winked at Georgia. He shifted the glasses on his nose. "Say, Marty, wanna see the rest of this place?"

Dale proudly displayed his handiwork. He had just poured a new concrete floor in their small garage. The summer before, he had built the little shed that housed their tools.

Their farmhouse, the dream of any city person tired of the rat race, was totally self-supporting. Dale explained the workings of a cistern to me. He told me that they used it to recycle rainwater for their washing machine.

Immediately adjacent to the wood frame house was an underground storm shelter stocked with canned goods and water. Out across the sprawling front lawn that led to the roadway stood the large vegetable garden that was Georgia's pride. Rows of corn, squash, green beans, and many other edibles stood ready for the summer harvest.

Finally, after Georgia and Dale excused themselves to go fix dinner, I set up my tent. I was inside preparing my sleeping bag when I heard Dale's voice outside.

"Hey, Marty, how 'bout a cold one?"

Dale asked me questions about my ride as we gazed out across the open fields drinking our beers. I congratulated myself on winning his friendship. In the past, when a situation involving other people had become difficult, I had just moved on to something else.

Soon, Georgia appeared with fruits and vegetables from her garden. After a few trips to the kitchen the picnic table was piled high with ears of corn and bowls filled with mashed potatoes, summer squash, and fresh-cut broccoli.

"Okay, dig in, you guys. Don't be bashful, Marty, just help yourself," Georgia commanded.

I felt like I was in heaven. I ate and ate. What made it even better was the fact that Georgia wouldn't let me stop.

"Go ahead, Marty. Let's go ahead and get it all finished," she said, as she passed a once-full plate of corn on the cob to me.

"I feel dumb. I've had what, about six already? I'm eating you out of house and home," I protested.

"I don't think that's going to be a problem," she said, smiling. She nodded over to her overflowing garden.

After I finished, Georgia handed me a big dish of fresh fruit. The assortment of blackberries, apple and peach slices, watermelon chunks, and raspberries tasted even better than it looked.

After we finished eating, we talked some more about my adventures. Then, as if a meal, a night's lodging, and a shower weren't enough, Georgia offered to wash my clothes.

"Aw, heck, Georgia, you don't have to do that." Of course she wouldn't take no for an answer.

When evening fell, I lay safe and warm in my little tent. I considered how blessed I'd been. Even though they would probably never see me again, Dale and Georgia had treated me like one of their own. A pile of clean laundry lay neatly folded next to the door of my tent, and I had enough fresh fruit to last me for days.

As I rolled my bike out to the road early the next day, a muffled voice called my name. I looked back at the house. Dale and Georgia were waving goodbye to me from their kitchen. As I put my legs in motion, I suddenly wished that I could turn back and express my gratitude better. Somehow mere thanks didn't seem enough. Their only request was that I let them know how I was doing with my ride. Georgia even gave me some address labels.

Later that day, I arrived in Danville, Illinois, at rush hour. I decided to wait it out at a gas station. A rusty pickup truck pulled in. A rough-looking man got out and walked over to the cashier. He said something, then they both looked over at me and started laughing.

A few moments later, he walked over toward me. He was a big man, and he was dressed in grease-stained pants. He wore a ripped denim jacket and thick-soled work boots. He looked like trouble.

My body stiffened. His scarred, hard face looked like it had seen many a bar room brawl. He stopped several feet from me, and his childlike words surprised me.

"You look like you could use some nice, juicy beefsteak tomatoes."

"Tomatoes?"

"Yeah, I growed 'em myself. Come on over to the truck."

"I'm not really into tomatoes," I said. Was this some kind of a trick? Maybe they were trying to lure me away from my bike so they could steal it. And if he did have tomatoes, how could I possibly know if they weren't spiked with some kind of poison? There were way too many reasons why I should stay away. But then I remembered that I had won many times before with people out here on the road when I had looked for the good in them.

"But if you grew 'em, let me take a look," I continued.

In the back of his truck was a little tricycle and a couple of shopping bags full of tomatoes.

"This is my kid's bike. I told Vern there that I was a gonna offer you a bag of tomatoes and this tricycle for your bike."

"Not fair," I laughed. I could see that he was a simple man whose rugged looks hid a gentle interior.

"But no, I came to bring you some beefsteaks, free of charge," he said. "I got a whole backyard full of 'em so I give 'em to people who look like they need them. Don't mind me; I'm just happy to be of service."

I took a few tomatoes and thanked him. I had misjudged this man badly. If I expected the worst from people, how could I expect them to do any better with me?

About an hour later, I crossed the state line into Indiana on Highway 32. The town of Perrysville, right on the border, could have fit into the glove box of the tomato man's truck. Cozy and rustic, its main block consisted of a handful of storefronts. The houses that surrounded the general store were not shielded from one another by fences. Instead, thick, green lawns grew from one property to the next.

I passed a small elementary school. The splotchy lawn that served as a part of its playground looked like it might make a comfortable bedroom floor. I biked a block past it into the main part of town and stopped at the general store.

Inside, a little bit of everything from plumbing supplies to sporting goods and grocery items greeted me. I searched around for a bread section only to find bicycle tires and model airplanes mixed in with canned goods and toilet plungers. The store's yellowish lighting shone down upon an inventory that seemed to date back to postwar years. More old items hung from the ceilings and walls.

I walked out the swinging doors with my loaf of bread. I knew its shelf life had been extended for many days by preservatives, but I needed something for my peanut butter sandwiches. Two little girls stood chattering near my bike.

I smiled at them. "Say, do you girls know if I can camp down in the school's park?"

They looked at one another, confused. "Why do you want to camp there?" the shorter one demanded. Her sandy hair, freckled face, and chubby little body set her apart from her tall, thin, dark-haired friend.

"I'm riding from California and I need a place to stay. That's why."

"Is that why you got so much stuff on your bike?" said the taller one.

They were of no help, and I was tired. "It was nice meeting you girls. I've got to head on down the road if I want to get my tent set up before it gets dark."

But they insisted on joining me in my ride back down to the park. So did one of their friends. Soon I found myself leading a convoy of little girls and their bikes through the small town. We exchanged names, and no sooner had we arrived than they excused themselves, promising to return.

While the little girls scurried off on their little Stingray bikes, I cleared rocks and pebbles from where my tent was to stand. Just as I got my camp stove going, a pickup truck rumbled into the schoolyard.

"Marty, we brought our dad to meet you!" one of the girls called from the truck.

Soon, the two girls I had first met, Susie and Laurie, stood before me with a smiling fellow they claimed was their dad. Unshaven and still dressed in his work clothes, he looked tired.

Usually, after a hard day's ride, my body also felt fatigued. I especially found it difficult to get myself moving and talking again after I had settled into a campsite. In fact, I tried to economize every movement and spoken word, and that was the case now. Looking up slowly from my dinner chores, I said, "Oh, hi. I've heard all about you from your girls. Nice to meet you."

I remained seated. Ron seemed to understand. He was a man of few words, so I broke up the silence with questions. We talked about Perrysville, his ex-wife, and his kids.

"Say, what happened to your friend Janet?" I asked the girls.

Susie answered. "Oh, her mom said that she had to stay home and eat dinner."

Ron seemed to have decided that I was a good guy. "How would you like to stay at our house tonight? It's not much, but we'd love to have ya."

I tried to find the right words to politely say no. I knew if I accepted his invitation I would wear myself down even more trying to earn my welcome.

"Gee... thanks a lot, Ron, but I can't even find enough energy to move. I've also got most of my camp already set up. I hate to, but I'm going to have to pass."

His daughters groaned in unison. "Aw, come on, Marty," they pleaded.

I looked at their drawn faces and began to weaken.

Laurie, the ponytailed, taller one, then piped in. "Oh, please, we don't have anything to do and we never saw a bicycle camper before. My dad says it's all right. Please?"

How could I contest that type of logic? Laurie and Susie were bored. They wanted someone to play bicycle with and had even gotten permission from their dad.

Ron made their request official. "Marty, we can just throw your bike in the back of the truck here." He just wanted to make his little girls happy. "It's only two blocks. I'm sure that Laurie and Susie would be happy to help pick up your things."

"Well... how 'bout if I just meet you guys down there. Let me collect my wits and I'll be down in a bit."

A short while later, I made it to their house. Even though Ron offered to sleep on the couch so that I could use his bed, I chose the soft lawn. As I set up my camp in their backyard, I heard Susie talking about me to her friends on the phone. I could also hear Laurie, the lady of the house, telling Susie who to call and what to say as she fixed a pancake dinner for all of us.

After pancakes, the four of us sat on the porch that overlooked their big yard and sipped iced tea, talked, and swatted mosquitoes.

Several years ago, Ron had left Perrysville with his wife for the sunny promise of California. He returned without her; he decided to raise his little girls in this wholesome environment. Both of them were straight "A" students. They also played on the school baseball team.

At nine o'clock, I excused myself to my tent. Susie and Laurie protested. They wanted me to stay up so they could learn more about me for their playmates.

"It's bedtime for you girls, too," said Ron. "Let's let Marty get some sleep. Good night, Marty."

All through the night, I heard the back door open and close. Later I would find out that Susie, who couldn't sleep, kept checking to make sure that I hadn't left without saying goodbye.

I awakened to the first light of the day and poked my head out of the tent to find my hosts already up. Little Laurie seemed to know the best way to a cyclist's heart, as pancakes were sizzling on the grill again. Somehow she knew that pancakes the night before did not mean that I wouldn't enjoy them as much the morning after.

Even though Susie's red eyes betrayed her lack of sleep, she, too, wanted to help in some way. So while Laurie cooked breakfast, Susie folded my ground tarp and the clothes they had washed for me.

Ron joined us for breakfast. Both of us ate quickly. While Ron had readied himself for his workday as a welder, I had prepared myself for the road.

"Well, I gotta hit it," I said as I brought my plate to the sink. "Those pancakes were great, Laurie, just about the best I ever tasted."

Laurie's smile was a wide one. "Marty, is it okay if me and my sister ride with you?'

As I walked to my bike, I asked, "Well, is it all right with your dad?"

Susie was quick to join in. "Oh yes, my dad says it's okay!"

I looked to Ron, who was standing by the back door. He nodded. What to do? I hoped they didn't want to ride with me for very long. As nice as they were, even half an hour could be unbearable. I like to get a good, strong start in the morning.

I decided to scare them. "Well, I don't know, you guys. It gets pretty hot out there, and you'll have to ride all the way back, tired and sore. I don't know."

Laurie laughed. "But we just want to ride with you to the bridge. It's not that far."

I felt tremendously relieved.

"Well... all right," I said as I straddled my waiting bike. "What are we waiting for, girls? Let's ride."

As Laurie and Susie hopped on their little bikes, Ron looked on approvingly. They rode on either side of me, flanking me like a touring general. As they rang their little bells, we rode off, headed for the Wabash River bridge.

"No farther than the bridge, now," Ron shouted as we disappeared from view. "Good luck, Marty."

I left Laurie and Susie on the town side of the bridge. They were still waving to me when I looked back just before rounding a corner out of sight.

Ron's blessing brought me even more hospitality in Indiana and Ohio. I enjoyed one day after the other of generously offered breakfast, lunch, and dinner at nearly every stop I made. Some of the Hoosiers and Buckeyes even gave me T-shirts and new farm caps in an attempt to outdo the hospitality that had preceded them.

In the more than two hundred miles between Perrysville, Indiana, and Chillicothe, Ohio, I shared meals with Ron the welder, a priest, a pig farmer and his family, two separate households full of schoolteachers, a graduate student and his wife, a bike shop owner, and a family at a picnic. This

Midwestern charm didn't really end until I reached the eastern part of Ohio and then crossed into West Virginia over the Ohio River.

Here, the hilly earth made it hard for anyone to make a living off the land. The evidence was everywhere: the older cars that rumbled along the winding roads and the ramshackle shacks and house trailers that began to appear on both sides.

Fortunately, once I crossed the Ohio River, Washington, D.C., was only a couple hundred miles worth of the Appalachian Mountains away. Once I had descended from the Rockies, I had relied on people for water, food, encouragement, and even a place to sleep at night. As fewer people populated the lands I now traveled through, I was glad to be nearing my destination. My body was stronger than ever, but the everyday wear and tear was exhausting me, and my upper back was in constant pain.

When I left home, I had been tired of people. I had come to think that they, not me, caused my inner pain. But I saw now how wrong I'd been. I needed them, and I promised myself never to think that I could do without them again.

The Appalachians proved no match for the Rocky or Sawtooth mountain ranges. As I roller-coastered through their eastern slopes, I became more and more excited. I wanted badly to prove to Dad and those who knew me that I could finish something. My sightseeing declined. I wanted to get to Washington, D.C., as fast as I could. I didn't let rain, fog, flat tires, a forty-mile-per-hour downhill crash, or the motorist who literally pushed me and my bike off the road stop me. I rode with a stronger purpose than ever.

The nation's capital was 138 miles away when I awoke one morning late in August. I felt like a well-oiled machine as my bike and I zoomed past the horse farms that stood alongside Highway 50. My legs felt like iron pistons. I tugged against the handlebars, pulling my body weight into the pedals as I pushed harder and harder. I refused to be distracted by roadside businesses.

That afternoon, for the first time in forty-five days, I saw smog. A blanket of brown haze covered my destination. Washington, D.C., suddenly did not seem as attractive as it once had. But I couldn't turn back. I had to finish.

A city stoplight. Parking lots. Concrete and steel as far as I could see. All of it had become foreign to me. Eugene,

Oregon, was the last big city I had ridden through. Since then, I had purposely steered as far away from population centers as I possibly could to avoid big city people and traffic, even when doing so had pulled me north or south.

At last I had to stop. A freeway made me. It separated me from my destination, the completion of my journey. Somewhere on the other side was D.C.

I was unprepared for this obstacle. My torn and tattered maps couldn't find a way around it. After 4,200 miles of deserts, mountains, and rivers, I was obstructed by a stretch of road that I couldn't enter.

I was suddenly weary, and anxious for my ride to end. I got a ride into the main part of town from a car. As soon as I got out and began pedaling toward the White House, I wondered when someone would notice who I was. I hoped that I would be besieged by autograph seekers and newspaper reporters as soon as someone found out what I had just done.

Nobody cared. They were too busy with their own lives. While the Midwestern farmers had made me the center of attention, here I was an absolute nobody.

Once again, the pain that I had felt at St. Alphonsus Hospital back in Boise began to overwhelm me. I wondered if the reception I had gotten back in the Midwest was even real. People here shook their heads as if they felt sorry for me and my road-weary bike.

I wanted to cry. Just because I didn't have a briefcase and wasn't neatly manicured with a trimmed beard and freshly pressed suit didn't mean that I was any less than the people that surrounded me. Only a few more blocks, I thought.

"Get a job," a cab driver shouted as I turned and held up traffic on a one-way street.

I nearly collapsed on the handlebars. How much more could I take? I looked at him, searching for some understanding. He gave me a nasty look and drove off.

The dark, gloomy sky poured down rain. Everyone scrambled for cover. By the time I reached the steps of the Capitol there were no onlookers to bear witness to my achievement. The rain shortened my celebration, and I pedaled to a nearby coffee shop.

Looking out the window at the Washington Monument, I began to think about home.

"What can I get you? It looks like you're a long way from home," the gray-haired waitress said.

"Just an orange juice, thanks." I was too depressed to give her any details.

I knew that she would be impressed with some of my tales from the road. But suddenly I realized that the only people I really cared about impressing were thousands of miles away. I felt lonelier than I ever had on the road.

What was so bad about the people I had left behind, anyway? The all-consuming challenge of the road had allowed me to forget why I had run away in the first place. Maybe they would see me as a different person if I went back. Maybe I could contribute to their lives like they had to mine when I'd needed them the most. But was I strong enough to be able to help others?

Maybe I could contribute by helping them to appreciate all that we take so much for granted. When I first got out of the hospital, I'd had great difficulty expressing that feeling. But I had developed the confidence to express my delight for even the simplest of things. I realized how self-centered, how selfish I'd been. It was then that I felt my rehabilitation was complete. I was eager to show Dad, and all the others who had helped me come back, that I was a new and improved Martin Krieg. I didn't realize how far I still had to go.

Looking out onto the rainy streets of the capital, I finally smiled. It had been a long journey.

Chapter 9

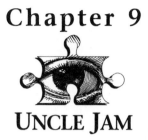

UNCLE JAM

The novelty of my achievement, at least for my family and friends, wore off in a few short weeks. They were busy trying to make their own lives work. They didn't seem to understand the enormity of what I had done. To most of them, it was just a bike ride, nothing more. "You gonna make your living riding bikes?" was my father's predictable response. He seemed to be almost embarrassed by my accomplishment.

After a day in D.C. I had started toward New York. But twenty miles out of Washington I got lost, and I just packed it in. Even though I hadn't planned on going back to the West Coast anytime soon, I found myself missing it and the people there. I packed my bike up and flew back to California the next day.

The story of my beating my car wreck with a transcontinental bike ride helped me sell my way back into the business field. But it didn't help me much once I got there. I could not hold on to any job. I was fired time and time again. Soon the bitter feelings that my car wreck had distanced me from began to surface.

Soon even those who I thought understood what I had just accomplished deserted me as well. The only person who wanted to take the time to help me was my Uncle Jim. I called him Jam because he was always rushing to get somewhere or trying to finish whatever he was doing as fast as he could.

"Hey, rookie, see the news today? Building new office building, downtown Oakland, probably need accountants," Jam said to me as he turned his road-worn six-cylinder Valiant through a corner gas station to avoid a red light. It was the summer of 1980, and we were on our way to umpire a baseball game in Oakland. I was living in San Leandro, and Jam had helped me get started umpiring in the area.

"You know I don't read newspapers or watch TV anymore.

I don't even listen to the radio. I just read self-improvement books. Besides, I told you, I don't want to be an accountant."

"Well... building a building doesn't just mean accounting jobs."

Jam was a borderline genius, but he had an odd habit of eliminating articles, prepositions, conjunctions, and other small words from his speech for the sake of economy. It sometimes sounded like some kind of advanced pidgin English and took some getting used to. He was a fit-looking guy in his late thirties, with a receding hairline and thick black-rimmed glasses.

Unlike most people, who would not wait for me to finish speaking, Jam never interrupted me though my words were slow. He remembered how well I'd done in school. He seemed to understand that an intelligent human being was behind the words that still came out haltingly.

"Well, don't know, rook. That's why you work with me as baseball umpire. Business suits are for automatons."

"Why'd you even bring it up then? Watch out for that milk truck." It surprised me how fast I had just spoken.

"See 'em. Go around." Jam turned to avoid the double-parked milk truck. "Son, you always tell me how you want convince family and friends that you're not loony. So I figure I whip out job you want so you can find out why ump better."

"It's not so much that, Jam. It's just that I want to get back in the mainstream. I thought that after I did my bike ride everyone would be impressed, but now they think I'm even weirder. That I don't fit in."

"Fuck 'em, rook, you can't be living for them."

"I don't know. Here I'm all proud that I proved those doctors wrong that wanted to amputate my leg, and instead I've got all my friends teasing me because they think my legs are too big."

"Jealous, rook. Kid stuff."

"What do you do? I mean, I want to get back to where I fit in and I can spend money on things like I used to when I was an accountant, and not always have to worry about where my next meal's gonna come from."

After more than two years my mind still had difficulty staying with one thought. It occasionally seemed to traipse off wherever it felt like.

Jam had paused to understand what I was trying to say.

"What's worst can happen, rook? You starve to death. Right?"

"I guess so."

"Well, rook. People don't starve to death in U.S. When last time you saw someone you know dying of starvation? People will always feed you. Get hungry, you can always get some food from friend or family member. Even if they don't like you, they won't let starve to death."

"I have a hard time getting respect ever since my car wreck."

Jam frowned as he considered this new admission.

"Gotta respect yourself first. Gotta love what you're doing, son. That's why I ump."

"Well, I don't think I want to ump the rest of my life. Who wants people yelling at you all the time?"

"Rook, you see 'em yelling at me? Just takes time. When you exude confidence in yourself, they won't rag on you."

"I don't know. It just seems like a thankless job. The more anonymous you are, the less you get noticed, the better you are. I don't know. Besides, I gotta spend time working on myself. I want to get all the way better."

"Look fine to me, son."

"That's just it, Jam. I may look fine, but I've still got a lot of things to work on. My dad makes fun of me for limping. He says I should have been working on walking instead of biking across the U.S. My face still droops, especially when I get tired. And I still get tired real easy. I have to take a pretty good nap if I'm going to do anything at night, like work these games. And I get interrupted all the time because I still talk too slow and sometimes I goof a lot of the words up."

"Stuff just takes time, rookie. You don't have to say much when you ump, what's the big deal?"

"It still pisses me off that I can't put a watch on without it being a big undertaking. Fastening the shirt buttons, like on this shirt, took me about ten minutes. I know that I'm a lot moodier than I ever was, too."

"What's ten minutes? I teach you how save that time on stoplights." Jam laughed. "You watch a lot of these people in hurry and they race up to one stoplight after another. And then what they do when get there? They wait for light turn green. Then fly off to next red light."

"So?" I knew I was guilty of the same crime.

"Waste more time in gas stations. Waste more time tune-ups, brakes."

"How else are you supposed to get there faster?"

"You read light, rookie. You see how I'm always studying traffic? I look ahead two, three intersection. Makes mind sharp. Keeps you from being automaton. Always gotta be thinking, not waste money, time."

"I've got all this education and I'm wasting it on baseball umpiring... there's no money in it, anyway."

Jam saw that as an opportunity to talk about one of his hobbies.

"Rookie, reach in the glove box there and try to find the coupon for free cookie at Loray's."

I opened the metal door. An envelope filled with coupons, pieces of paper, newspaper articles, and schedules and addresses spilled out. A baseball rolled out and landed on the boxes that my feet straddled on the floor.

"Jam, I don't want to look through all this junk for a free cookie."

"Look for cookie. Stay free. That's how we work system, rook. You take time to save coin, otherwise you do something you no like, to make coin. The Jam show you how live off the land."

"But that's what I mean, Jam. Everyone thinks I'm weird already. I'm not gonna go around redeeming coupons. I used to make good money as an accountant."

"But what else you do, rook? Did you get sunshine, fresh air?"

"On weekends. No, but I had respect and I could buy what I wanted to buy."

"Where things now, rookie?"

"I just finished with the bike ride and you know I sold everything."

"That's what I mean. You sold it all so you could do what you want. I do what I want all time. Rook, we're almost there, help me get the rest of this chest protector on. You work plate first game tomorrow, I work plate this game."

"You're gonna put your shirt over this while you're driving?"

"Son, all the time."

"No, what I mean is this," I said as I snapped the clips on Jam's chest protector. "My family thinks I'm a real bum hanging out with you umpiring baseball games."

"Rookie son," Jam cackled, "worry about what everyone else thinks, you never free. Do you want to do other people's job's just so you can be liked or do you want do what you want do?"

"Who says I want to umpire?"

"You no make coin old way because bike ride now show you what important, right? It show you want to be in sunshine breathing fresh air. It show you that you no want be dull normal inside office all day shuffling papers."

Uncle Jam never teased me for my inability to hold down a job. He was trying to tell me that there was more to life than just blindly following a career path just for the sake of making money.

"But I've got all these friends and family that really think I'm blowing it."

"Screw 'em, rookie, you gotta figure what you want, not what they want. We get you sharp. We get you thinking on your feet. Bike ride took you out of automatic, but now we got make sure you no return to dull normal habits."

As we traveled from game to game, sometimes in as many as five different ballparks in a day, Uncle Jam and I discussed many of life's dilemmas in this way. I had naively thought my bike ride would inspire everyone. Instead, it had only increased the distance between myself and my family and friends. It made me even more different. It made it even more difficult for them to try to relate to my life, especially when I refused to rejoin the rat race.

Uncle Jam was the only one who seemed to understand me—maybe because he had been ostracized from the family because he chose to live outside of the system. A college dropout, he had once supported himself by taking tests and writing papers for other students for a fee. I had always been fascinated by Jam. He could have had it all. At one time, he had been pursued by pro scouts to play professional baseball. Back then he seemed to be enjoying the company of a different beauty queen every time I saw him. That sure got my attention.

He was blessed with great athletic ability and a quick mind. But the system bored him. He wanted to feel challenged. So now Uncle Jam worked half of the year umpiring high school, college, semipro, and city league baseball games. He squirreled away his money so he could spend the other half of his year learning from books. His image wasn't enhanced by the fact that he lived at his ninety-year-old grandmother's house.

We finally arrived at the ballpark where we were scheduled to work.

"I got to get some new slacks," I said, brushing my ump slacks off as I climbed out of the car. I only owned one pair for umpiring.

Both teams and their fans stared at us as we walked from the parking lot to join them.

"Rookie, more slavery, no need new slacks. We do garage sales tomorrow. Recycle time. Cost you fifty cents."

"I don't want to wear someone else's pants."

"Rookie, dull normal buys pair of pants, wears two time and then he sells for quarter. Sometimes they no fit and you get pair he too lazy to take back. We'll get pair tomorrow. Let's whip, son."

"It's about time, you guys," said one of the coaches.

"What time you got?" Jam asked.

"Two-fifty-eight."

"Let's play ball," shouted Jam, and briskly walked to home plate. Jam always wore the baggiest jackets and shirts that he could find. It was all I could do to keep from laughing the first few times we umpired baseball games together. Dressed in the second-hand clothes that were usually given to him by one of his uncles, he looked more like a street person than an umpire.

"What took you guys so long?" the coach from the other team said as he handed over the lineup card.

"Traffic," Jam said with a straight face. We could hear the coach muttering as he walked away shaking his head.

"We could have been here ten minutes earlier if you hadn't stopped and taken your time to pick out a watermelon," I said under my breath.

"Game starts at three, I'm here at three. They no pay us to be here any earlier. Besides, can't miss watermelon on sale. Don't waste gas, rook. Combine trips."

"We could have left fifteen minutes earlier, then."

"For a baseball game? Rooookiie... " Jam laughed.

I didn't always agree with Jam's approach to life. Sometimes I relied on the teachings in my books to get through some of the more embarrassing times that he would put me through. I found myself continually challenged to know which of his teachings I needed to hang on to and which I should throw out the window.

"Second base," said Jam. I took my cue and ran to my

position behind the first baseman. The catcher took the last warm-up throw and fired the ball to the shortstop standing over second base.

"Let's have a batter!" Jam bellowed.

And with that the game began.

"Who's the new blue?" One of the kids asked Jam as he walked from the on-deck circle.

"That's the rookie, we'll break him in," Jam responded.

The kids, all college age, seemed to like Jam. Many of the players from both teams carried on a brief dialogue with him every time they came to bat. They clearly knew of his past successes as a baseball player.

As the game wore on, several close calls challenged my ability to make instantaneous decisions. Between innings, Jam and I talked about it.

"Rook, you got to sell your calls. These coaches think that because I'm late that I bring along stooge who can't make right calls. Your calls look right, you're just not selling them, son."

"What do you mean?"

"You can't pause more than second. Makes it look like you're not sure. Also, close call at first or like that one at second, you let the whole ballpark know about it. Especially on tag plays at second because you're so far away, they can't see anything anyway. Just remember, rook, when in doubt call 'em out. Outs make game go faster. Don't worry about blowing it, I'll cover for ya."

Jam helped me overcome my nervousness my first few games like that. He knew that I would make mistakes but he had confidence in his own ability as an umpire to keep the game under control. Jam was able to keep the purpose of the game in perspective. He tried to make sure the players all had fun, and if one of my calls caused an unfavorable reaction, he reminded the injured party as diplomatically as possible that we were only playing a game.

"But Jam, you know I'm still working on getting my voice to go louder."

"Practice with your out calls. Batter up!"

When the game ended, the losing coach came up and congratulated Jam. "Thanks for a good game. Sorry I gave you a bad time for being late. The kids really love having you do their games."

"Thanks, coach. We got to whip," Jam returned as he

collected his gear and started walking off the diamond. We talked baseball and life as we drove back to my house in his Valiant.

"Time, rookie? Want to know how long game took us."

"Six-thirty. Why don't you wear a watch?"

"What, wear a little machine on arm?" Jam snickered. "I let you do that."

"What do you do when I'm not around?"

"Come on... easy to get within fifteen minutes by looking at where sun at in sky. You look at where shadows fall. Kind of like Indians always know what time without needing little machines. Indian not disconnected from day. Indian live off land. No need clocks, rook. Man invented clock, not nature."

"Okay, but what if I'm not here and you need to know exactly what time a game started, like today?"

"Just ask somebody."

"But what if there's nobody around?"

"If no one around, time doesn't matter, does it, son?"

"Okay... what if you're in a car, and you have to be somewhere?"

"You look around. Anywhere there's people, gonna be clocks. You look inside store windows. They have 'em on buildings. Live in city, clocks everywhere. Live in country, clock is sun."

Jam questioned every value or belief system that I had in this way. By refusing to allow me to accept even the simplest of life's absolutes, Jam tried to sharpen my dulled mind.

"How was my game?" I was tired of talking about the time of day.

"You're getting better, rookie. That one call of yours down at second could have gone either way. You could have sold safe also," Jam said as he sped up a freeway on-ramp.

"I just remembered what you said, my head was bouncing up and down as I ran to get there and I know I wasn't in position yet, so I just called 'out' as loud as I could."

"All right. You'll learn position in time, just always remember they're not paying to call safe. Pussies call safe because that's the easy way. Gotta be strong to call somebody out."

"What time do we start tomorrow, anyway?"

"Eight o'clock. Two-fourteen Taylor."

"You want me to be at your house at eight? I thought games didn't start on Saturday before ten."

"They don't, but we got garage sale duty."

"Jam, I told you, I don't want to buy anything at a garage sale. I'd rather wait till I get a real job and can buy the stuff new."

"What, you want fancy plastic bag with store name on it? I get new stuff all time at garage sales," Jam said as he nodded toward his cluttered back seat.

A catcher's mitt lay on top of a pile of board games, a down vest, soccer cleats, baseball cards, candy wrappers, and spark plug wires.

"But this stuff ain't new. Looks like a bunch of junk."

"Most people think like you do. That's why no one steals it. Be resourceful, rook, there's all kinds of great stuff in there. And it's hardly used. But it might have someone else's germs on it, son. That whole back seat cost me maybe pocket of change. What, are you too proud?"

We pulled up in front of my house. It had been a long day of umpiring, four games in all. As Jam pulled away, he yelled, "Two-fourteen Taylor, eight o'clock, whip, whip!"

I was too tired to shower. I collapsed onto my bed and fell asleep immediately.

The next morning I rode my bike the ten miles from my house to Alameda, where Jam lived. I leaned my bike against the steps and knocked on the door.

His old Italian grandmother answered. She was bent over at the waist, and her long gray hair was pinned on top of her head in a bun. A black cat ran out the door.

"Aaaah, that cat, he scared. You wanta Jimmy, I get a broom that lazy bum," she said in a thick Italian accent. "He and Joe they two bums. All they do is sleep."

Joe was Grandma's sixty-five-year-old son who had never left the house. He worked as a school janitor and drove the same car he had owned as a teenager.

"You go and wake. I no want that bum sleep all a the time."

I knocked on his bedroom door and walked in.

"Get up, Jam, you told me eight o'clock."

"Rookie alarm clock service here. Let's whip." Jam stretched. "Get newspaper from Grandma."

I obediently returned with the newspaper. Without a word Jam started marking up the garage sale section with a magic marker.

"What are you doing?"

"Gotta have a plan. We do whole island. Take forty-five-minute with plan," Jam grabbed a notebook and started plotting the codes to a grid he had drawn to represent the major streets of Alameda.

"It takes almost that long to drive around it in a car."

"Let's whip, rook, that's what I mean. You navigate and I'll get us to all, let me count 'em," Jam paused as he added the numbers up, "twenty-two garage sales today. I can size 'em up in two seconds."

"What do you mean?"

"We find garage sale rookies who just want to clear out their garage. We stay away from ones who want make money off poor umpires."

"How are we supposed to do that?"

"If they've got the stuff all organized and look like they took lot time to set up, those people charge more. You offer them dime for something and if they go crazy, we move on. Also, we stay away from garage sales where they have the prices on little tags. How stupid. You'll see these goofy people go out and buy these little tags to put price on so they don't forget. They get to play department store for day."

"Aren't you embarrassed to offer someone a dime for something?"

"It's just a token, rook, if they just want to lighten their load, they figure you paid the price of embarrassing yourself with that kind of offer. Try it. I never pay more than twenty-five cents for anything. If one sale don't let you have it for that, another one will. Might not even be that day. Might even take a summer to find that price. But that's half the fun. Call it marking time. Makes you appreciate more."

Jam collected his things and we dashed out the door to his car.

"You man the list, rook," Jam said as we turned on to a long tree-lined boulevard. "We're on Central now, what the first one you got there?"

"Eight-ninety. You mean to tell me I might have to wait all summer for another pair of slacks for umpiring?"

"Three more lights—whip! You can wait all summer or you can spend all your time under fluorescent lights and buy twenty pairs that you never get time to wear. Good ump know how mark time. No hurry. More laundry till find. Challenge."

"Then don't you forget you wanted certain things?'

"If you forget, then you no need. Everyone wants you to buy things so they can lock you into mainstream. Your family wants you buy new things so you'll have to keep doing stuff to make them happy and not you. That's how system works. I'm showing you how to stay out of system."

Even though I desperately wanted to be accepted by the system and those already in it, Jam's challenge was seductive. I began to look for ways to improve on his methods. I started keeping lists. My self-improvement books said that if you wrote something down, you moved yourself that much closer to its attainment. Not only could I improve my penmanship, list-keeping also freed my mind to think about other things.

I also began to see garage sales as a way to improve my dexterity. I still found myself struggling with watchbands, shirt buttons, and all sorts of other skills involving manual dexterity. Even the baseball clicker I used to keep track of balls, strikes, and outs gave me problems. I knew I needed wintertime projects that would help me fine-tune my coordination deficiencies.

"What do you want that for, rook, it's missing half of its parts," said Jam one day later that summer. We were at a garage sale, and I was looking at a bike.

"I can take the racks off and put 'em on my three-speed."

"Ask them for the racks, then."

"No, I want the whole bike, it's got a good frame and I can build it up over the winter with parts from all these other bikes I've been scoring."

"You're just gonna make your landlady even madder you keep bringing these things home. You've already got a stack of 'em behind metal shed you built her."

"I just like to have a bunch of bikes around so people can come over and we can ride down to the marina and stuff. I'm probably going to ref basketball this winter, Brown thinks he can get me on, so I'll have the days free to get those bikes all running good."

I was living in a converted garage apartment. By the end of the summer it was filled with second-hand treasures. I bought junky bikes, motorcycles, and even cars, and fixed them up and sold them. Sometimes I'd make a couple hundred bucks, sometimes a lot less. But it kept me occupied, got me some extra money, and was great therapy for my motor skills.

Just as Jam had predicted, by marking time I had outfitted my little home with lamps, dishes, blenders, end tables, and many other amenities. I'd owned the same kind of stuff before, but I'd sold it all to finance my TransAmerica bike ride. But this stuff I'd bought with little more than a pocket full of change.

Whenever I spent a dime to cross a nutcracker, wine opener, dish rack, or coffee mug off my list, not only did I experience the thrill of accomplishment, but I reinforced my understanding of the temporary nature of things. Once I realized that I didn't have to work so hard to acquire the money to buy the things I thought I needed, I discovered that I could let them go a lot easier. This new feeling of freedom was enhanced when I found I could buy an almost-new blender, a down jacket, or a pair of shoes for a dollar if I just had some patience. After a while, this abstinence from impulse, along with my diligent list-keeping, made me feel like a rich man.

Garage sales were also therapy for me. They taught me how I could fit in with others by doing a better job of selling myself. They showed me that everything we do involves salesmanship in one way or another. Even as the buyer, I discovered that if I took a genuine interest in the seller or at least made the exchange fun for him, I could expect to get a bargain. And my garage sale successes reminded me of the interpersonal victories I had enjoyed on my bike ride across America.

"Mime Troupe Berkeley, free, one o'clock," Uncle Jam's voice at the other end of the phone greeted me one morning.

"What do mean, Mime Troupe?"

"Comedy, rook, Mime Troupe play Berkeley, beeeg time, half off co-ops, too."

"I don't want to sit around in the car while you hustle for half-priced food."

"Read walls then, son, while I score half-priced cheese and grapes and stuff they put out. You can read the classified wall they got. Bicycle parts, rook."

Jam had shown me the ads that the co-op stores let people post for free on one of their walls. Our regular trips to Berkeley also meant that I could pick up the free newspapers at the coffee shops, book cafes, and music stores. Many of the papers contained pages of classified ads. Not only did I often find great deals on bicycle parts but "reading the walls," as Jam phrased it, helped me to understand the latest trends in society.

I watched the computer revolution unfold as more and more people offered their services as instructors in this field. I saw the gay population gain acceptance as greater numbers of their ads requesting housing and relationships began to appear. I stayed current on the latest craze in entertainment by noticing which events people were scalping tickets for.

"Well, all right, you talked me into it."

As we sped down Telegraph Avenue in Berkeley that afternoon, Jam expounded on his traffic light strategy.

"See that light two intersections ahead? It just turned red, so that means if we waste gas trying to whip this one, then we're gonna have to stop right away anyway. So what I do is slow down and try time that one so we can pick up next one and one after that when they turn green. Don't be a victim, rook. Always drive three lights ahead. Makes you sharp."

"Who wants to always have to be reading lights when they drive? What about other traffic? I don't think it's such a safe thing to do."

"Becomes automatic, son. Beeeg time. Makes you sharp. Better in traffic because you're more alert, you're keen. You don't get lulled to sleep like most of these drivers out here, you're like an animal, always ready to react."

After an afternoon of bargain hunting and the Mime Troupe's political satire, which everyone seemed to understand but me, Jam and I headed home.

"Happy hour stop, rookie. Croll's has umpire food," Jam announced.

"Jam, I don't feel right about ordering water and eating up all their food. Besides, I don't think it's good to be eating leftovers all the time."

"You call chicken wings leftovers? I've seen 'em have guacamole and chips and other stuff, too."

"Yeah, but you can't live on that stuff."

"Who says? " Jam flexed his biceps.

We parked and went inside. Photos of sports stars looked down upon a brass-railed bar and mahogany tables filled with happy hour drinkers. One of the faces on the walls stood out from the rest.

"Who's that?" I asked.

"Rookie... " Jam shook his head sadly. "That's Jack London."

"Who's that?"

"He was a world-famous writer. You know, *Call of the Wild*? *White Fang*? You used to like him when you were a kid... must've been the car wreck. He used to hang out near the Oakland Estuary. All of his stories are real. He didn't make any of his stuff up. Lived all of them. He wasn't like a lot of these writers you get now, just do it safe way. They hide behind these little typewriters and make up stories about what they think it might have been like. Jack London was the real thing."

I had thought of writers in the same way. I had never before thought that an author could graduate from the working class, that our stories, no matter how unique, were anything that people would be interested in reading.

"He just wrote about regular stuff?"

"Jack London was a regular guy who wrote himself out of the factories. Just kept collecting rejection slips until his work started to sell. Wrote something like a thousand words a day, all by hand. They say he got to a point where he could write something one time and it was ready to go."

"I should write my story. I've had people tell me I should, but I never thought I was educated enough to be a writer."

Jam looked at me. "Son, I've heard that too much education can be problem for writer. They say you want be able write in way that reduces complex thoughts to simplest form."

"I can do that. I've got an incredible story to tell."

"Do it then, rookie."

Soon after I had moved into my converted chicken coop in San Leandro, there had been a knock on my door one afternoon. It was the San Leandro Chamber of Commerce Welcome Wagon, in the person of a bubbly, cheerful woman named Renata. We hit it off and got to talking, and I told her about my accident and ride. She encouraged me to write about my experiences and told me she was writing a book of her own. She recommended that I take some adult-education classes to improve my writing. We became good friends.

During the winter months, I hardly saw Jam as he went into self-imposed hibernation. I had more time to myself. I made a few undisciplined attempts to write my book. But I was easily distracted, and soon I began to spend a lot of time in a weight-lifting gym.

There I met Angie, who befriended me and helped me with my weight-lifting. Angie was a middle-aged man who was slightly shorter than me but twice as thick and a half again as wide. He helped me overcome the intimidation I initially experienced. He became another of my mentors. Handsome with a head of thick black hair, Angie had spent the greater part of his life working out in health clubs.

"I feel weird looking at myself in the mirror all the time," I said to Angie one day as I lifted a dumbbell on to a bench. The weight was far less than what I saw those around me using, but it still nearly pulled me over.

What I saw in the mirror continually reminded me of how much work I had yet to do. It embarrassed me to take my shirt off anywhere in public, especially here. I had a sunken chest, disproportionately large stomach, and skinny, T-shirt-tanned arms. That was a contrast with the lower half of my body, which ballooned out of my gym shorts. My bike riding had built huge masses of muscle into my legs, but it had done nothing for the upper part of my torso. It did show me that if I remained disciplined, in time I could expect to look and lift like the gym monsters all around me. I also knew that, just like my bike ride, the hardest part was getting started.

"That's the problem with the world today, Marty," Angie said, "you get these damn people who just don't like themselves. They've never taken the damn time to love themselves. So they don't like to see their bodies in the mirror."

"I love myself."

"That's what they all say. If you loved yourself, you wouldn't have a problem looking at yourself in the mirror. I'm talking about the whole person. Not just that face you see in your bathroom mirror. You're not a just a mind with a body attached, for cryin' out loud."

"I don't get it."

"That's the root, don't you see, Marty?" Angie could become quite passionate about the subject. "You gotta be able to like seeing all of the person that you see in the mirror. All these people that say we're a bunch of egotistical bastards are the same people that go out and kill and steal and every other damn thing. How can they respect or love others if they don't respect or love all of themselves first? And this is the place to start. Right there in the mirror.

What you see is how you judge yourself throughout the day. If you like what you see..."

"Is Angie lecturing you?" David, one of the gym's more developed bodybuilders, teased as he walked by on his way to the scale.

"Nah, he's probably telling me everything I need to hear," I answered.

"Well, you let me know if you need any help. Take care, Angie, I'm outta here."

I turned back toward Angie. "But what about what my dad means when he says that the meek shall inherit the earth?"

"Who says you can't be meek and take the time to love yourself? You can have it all if you love yourself. But you've got to be able to love yourself first before you can be meek enough to accept others with all of their faults, I'll tell ya. You see these little pencil-neck guys all the time, they're always the first ones to start a fight or criticize somebody for something. And that's because they just don't accept their damn selves. You know, Marty, when you realize that without you, there ain't gonna be no bills or girls or jobs or your dad to worry about, then you'll feel a little bit better about taking time to take care of yourself."

"I don't know, Angie, I'm only doing this till I get all the way better."

Angie and I had talked about my car wreck before. And he had given me many tips on how to overcome the right-sided strength deficiencies that I was still experiencing. He was, however, disappointed to hear that I had not planned to make body building a way of life.

"That's exactly what I'm talking about. You deserve to look great and feel great all the time. Your most important wealth is your health, Marty. Health is wealth." Angie liked to repeat this line over and over again. "You know, Marty, you tell me what you got without your health. You don't have anything. This is number one. Not all these fancy cars you see these kids slaving away for so they can drive them around. Health is more important than your business career. It's more important than anything. Hell, you can't enjoy all the money in the world without your health. Your accident should have shown you that."

"Yeah, but Angie, I want to prove to people that my life was worth saving."

"You prove that by loving yourself enough to give yourself the kind of time it takes to feel complete. Hell, I'm in this place two, three hours a day, every day. Been doing this for over thirty-five years, Marty. Do I look like other people my age that are all beaten into the ground by all these things that they think are so important, like bills, and cars, and houses?"

I looked at Angie's well-developed torso. It practically exploded out of his ripped sweatshirt. His strong Indian-like features added authority to his words.

"Hell, I've got everything that I see all these people losing their health over and then some. You've seen my cars. And hell, Marty, I live in a beautiful home and I've got two kids who respect and love me because I respect and love myself. What more can a guy ask for? All you're doing is taking care of what God gave you, aren't you? Think about it that way."

It made sense if you thought about it that way. And as the winter wore on, I became more and more addicted to the gym. A friend had crashed and destroyed my Eisentraut, and I had bought an old three-speed and fixed it up. I got up at six and biked three miles to the gym. Along the way, as I waved to the regulars along my route, I often dreamed of what it would be like to build an organization in which everybody biked to work. Bicycling seemed to be picking up momentum and converts. Would it ever reach that point?

My weights increased, and I began to see changes in my body. And I started to notice a new confidence in myself in almost all areas of my life. My TransAmerica bike ride was no longer the only reference point for my improvement. That seemed eons ago. Now I gauged my progress against chrome-plated dumbbells.

Since weight-lifting was a lifestyle, as Angie had pointed out, I also found myself interested in new ways of nourishing myself. I knew that I could not rely on the strength of youth to forever shield me from the harmful effects of junk food. One day, as I held a frozen yogurt in one hand and a well-used handkerchief in the other, a bike rider I had recently befriended told me about a new way to eat.

"You wouldn't be blowing your nose all the time if you ate right," Eli said as we stood on the corner facing Sproul Plaza at UC Berkeley.

Eli was a man of average height who spoke in clipped sentences. He had piercing eyes. Even though I knew he didn't work out, he still looked healthy and strong.

"I just didn't cover up after I left the gym today, that's all," I said dismissively.

"Not true," he stated. The tone of his voice and the clarity in his eyes told me his knowledge was based on experience.

"What do you mean, not true? I leave this hot gym and I don't cover up my throat and arms and I bike home, that's what gets me sick."

"Sure, you should cover up like that. But look what you got in your hand there."

"Yogurt. It's healthy."

"Yogurt. It's dairy."

"I know it's dairy. So what?"

"Did you know that cow milk is meant to fatten up a two-thousand-pound animal? Did you know that man is the only animal that drinks milk after he is weaned? The carbohydrate-to-protein ratio of mother's milk is seven to one. For cow's milk it's something like twenty-seven to one."

Eli reeled off these facts as if he had memorized them for a school play.

"How come they say milk does a body good, then?"

"Come on, Marty, are you serious? Do you believe everything you hear or read? Even worse than that, you believe commercials where people are paid to say what they say? A lot of black people can't even digest milk because they're lactose-deficient. Maybe that should tell you something. Ice cream is even worse. It's got four things going against it. It's cold, you should always avoid extremes. It's sweetened with the kind of simple sugars that confuse your pancreas. It's dairy, and a lot of it's even got preservatives in it that you find in paint thinners and such."

"How do you know all this stuff?"

"I used to live in a macrobiotic study house, back in Boston."

"You mean if I stop doing yogurt, I'll stop dripping at the nose?"

"I guarantee I can show you how to get rid of almost every symptom with proper diet."

"I'm sure," I said sarcastically.

"Do you know what Hippocrates, the father of medicine,

said? He said, 'let food be your medicine and medicine be your food.'"

I could see that Eli knew a lot. His confidence almost seemed cocky. I decided to test him.

"What do you eat for a cold then?"

"It's what you don't eat. You've got a yin condition. Yin, which is acid, means that you don't keep fueling the fire by putting more acid in it like orange juice. I find it humorous when people tell me they've been drinking lots of orange juice for their cold. Colds are also a mucus condition, so you don't keep adding mucus-forming foods—especially like milk."

"What's left, then?"

"How about root vegetables, like carrots and onions and burdock root in a mugi miso soup, for starters?"

"What do you eat?"

"I eat lots of brown rice."

"Brown rice?"

"Oh yes, it's a very important part of the macrobiotic diet. Brown rice is a perfectly balanced food. I eat two to three pressure cookers full a week."

"Pressure cooked?"

Eli started to smile. He knew he had aroused my curiosity. My head was beginning to spin with all this new information.

"I can put you on a food program where your sense of smell will return, you'll wake up every morning feeling great, and your colds and flus will become almost nonexistent."

"And what is that?"

"Macrobiotics. You won't believe what it will do for your endurance, also. You'll be able to bike forever if you eat macrobiotically."

"I don't know, Eli... it sounds like a lot of rules about what you can't eat."

"That's not true. In fact, you'll find out about foods that you never knew existed, like daikon, tempeh, wakame, miso. Have you ever heard of any of those?"

"If this stuff is so great, how come I've never heard of macrobiotics?"

"Because no one can make any money off it. All that macro is is eating simply and in balance. It's the oldest eating discipline known to man. It's centuries old and comes from the monasteries of Tibet. There are several excellent books about it, which I highly recommend you read."

That was all I needed to hear. I began to read everything
I could find about nutrition, and I compared the findings in
all of the regimens I found with the macrobiotic way. As I
applied what I was learning to my own life, Eli's words
about achieving optimal health seemed truer every day.

As soon as I retrained my taste buds away from the sugar
that I now knew was damaging me, I found myself hooked
on brown rice, vegetables, and miso.

My simplified diet and lifestyle, free of the sugars, meats,
and preservatives that my body had once worked overtime
to process, also sparked in me a curiosity about the spirit
realms. Books on spirituality replaced the steady diet of self-
improvement reading I had fed myself ever since my car
wreck. By the time my next season of baseball umpiring
arrived, I had even taught myself my own form of
meditation.

I had just returned to my garage apartment from the
gym one day the next spring when Karen, an attractive
woman I had begun to take an interest in, stopped by.

"Hi, Marty," Karen said as I opened the front door. "I was
just in the area, and I thought I'd stop by and say hello."

Karen was a freckle-faced blonde, and very intelligent.
She had just graduated from UC Berkeley with a degree in
anthropology. She was pretty close to the girl of my dreams.
She had long, straight, luxurious hair, and a tan and slender
body. I had met her at a wedding. She was working at a
restaurant nearby.

"I was going to meditate in a little bit, but I think I can
move that back just a little," I said, waving her in.

"Meditate? Don't you have to have some guru train you
for that or something?"

"That's what I used to think. Based on all the books I can
find about it, meditation is no more than a deep form of
relaxation. Kind of like where you allow yourself to be
released from the world and all its thoughts and distractions."

"What kind of distractions?"

"Well, TV and radio, to begin with. I even unplug the
phone. Then, as you start just letting yourself go, you have
to train yourself to empty your mind of any thoughts.
Because those are distractions, too."

She nodded. "How'd you learn to do it, anyway?"

"It's not that big a deal. I just combined what I had read

about Silva Mind Control, transcendental meditation, and some other books."

A walnut fell from a tree outside and landed loudly on the shed.

"I'm curious. What do you do when you do it?" Karen's almond-shaped eyes seemed to be inviting me to share my deepest thoughts with her.

"Well, first of all I make an appointment with myself, just like I schedule baseball games, the gym, or garage sales. I set aside an uninterrupted hour every day. Sometimes I have to break it up into half-hour chunks."

"Then what do you do?"

"You sure you want to hear? I mean, hey, this might sound weird."

"No, really... it sounds interesting."

"Well okay... I dim my bedroom by closing the curtains. I make sure the telephone is unplugged, like I said. Then I lie on my bed with my palms facing upward and adjust my body and head so that they're comfortable."

"Are you lying on your back?"

"Right. Then, I close my eyes and I breathe through my nose. You know, I couldn't breathe real good through my nose till I got off dairy and sugar and meat."

"Really? Okay, then what happens?" Karen's curiosity was disarming, and very exciting.

"I just let go and let my mind go where it wants to. But before I do that, I pray that God will take me to His world. Sometimes I just try to concentrate on my breath as it passes over my nose hairs to get me focused a little bit."

"Where do you go?"

"I don't know... I just feel rejuvenated and more at peace with myself. My problems, like where I'm gonna get next month's rent and stuff, don't seem as big. It's kind of like I'm going and getting help and I don't even know what they're doing for me. But it always seems to work. I even asked 'em to introduce me to somebody like you. Then I let it go, and look what they found."

She smiled. "You don't really believe that, do you?"

Several weeks later, Karen moved in with me.

Chapter 10

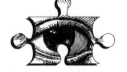

ANOTHER CROSSING

"Renata, thanks for calling back. I was just wondering… Have you talked to Marty lately?"

"Karen, it's been about, oh, a week ago. Would you believe he's living in a bomb shelter?"

"No, but that sounds like Marty. A bomb shelter as in World War II? Like a bunker?"

The older woman laughed. *"No, as in air raid shelter. It's in the basement of a mansion outside of town that was once a psychiatric hospital. It's now the recreation hall for an apartment complex. He's under the pool hall."*

Karen sighed. *"Sounds awful… is he doing okay?"*

"Oh, I think so. You know Marty, always living on the edge. The magazine folded, so he's back to working baseball and basketball games."

"Poor Marty. I just couldn't do it anymore, Renata. I loved him, but that book he was writing about his comeback was becoming this monster. It consumed all the money we had. I still think it's a great story. I mean, he could've spent the rest of his life in an institution. But so many things went wrong. You were around when he was writing it all out by hand. He even told me he was doing it that way because he read that was how his hero, Jack London, did it. But it was taking him forever. Then I persuaded him to type it, then he got it typeset when it needed editing first. Finally he bought that used computer and it took him months to key it in with all those changes that editor made. And then just after he finished, that damn machine destroyed it. That was the final straw. That depressed him so much that he was impossible to live with. I don't know if he's ever going to finish it now."

"You know how Marty is when he gets obsessed about something. That's all that exists in the world for him, and that includes people who love him. He doesn't have time for anybody else when he gets in that mode."

"I hope he gets over it… he can be so sweet when he wants to. He was the one who made me realize I had enough confidence to

manage the restaurant, you know." Her voice softened. "I miss him… but I just couldn't live like that anymore."

Karen was a breath of fresh air in my life. She was pretty, wonderful, smart, funny… I was crazy about her, and she said she was about me, too.

We lived together for almost three years. For a long time it was idyllic, even though my tiny converted garage had only four rooms. The small kitchen looked out on the landlady's neatly groomed backyard. A tiny bathroom housed a toilet and a compact sink and shower. The water pressure for both rooms depended on who was using what. Karen could not wash dishes while I showered, and we couldn't get water at all if the landlady was using hers. We slept on the foldout couch in the living room, and the last tiny room was my office.

Because she knew my family, she already knew about my accident, and my TransAmerica trip, and that I'd been planning on writing a book about my experiences. I'd been writing it out longhand, to practice my dexterity, but it was taking forever. I hadn't really taken it seriously until Karen persuaded me that it was a wonderful story that would make a great book. Her enthusiasm was infectious. Then she got me an old manual typewriter to type it on. I put my bike up on rollers, and I'd get up at five and turn on a self-improvement tape and ride for half an hour to get both my physical and mental juices going. Then I'd work on the typewriter until Karen came home from her waitressing job. At first you could hardly read it, there were so many typos, but I slowly got better.

But I was becoming arrogant about my story. Karen suggested an agent, then a librarian friend suggested an editor, but I didn't have any luck with the few agents I talked to, and I didn't have the money for an editor. I didn't think my writing was that bad, either. I was sure that if I just got it looking like a book that all the agents and publishers and producers and investors would be beating down my door to get a piece of my story. Nobody could tell me anything, least of all Karen. She even stuck by me after I insisted on getting it typeset so it looked more like a real book before an editor even looked at it, and when I bought a used Apple computer from a Berkeley student for $600 and started inputting my book.

I finally got it edited professionally. That showed me I had a lot of work to do to be a writer. I became consumed with getting better. I studied books and magazines like *Writer's Digest*, and took some adult education classes. I began writing and submitting stories to different magazines. I'd write in the morning, then go for long bike rides in the afternoon in the Oakland hills trying to figure out what I had to do to interest agents and publishers. I'd take inspiration from the thought of Jack London riding his high-wheel, bone-shaker bicycle the forty miles from Oakland to San Jose regularly. If he could do that, I could do anything.

Finally *Bicycling* magazine took one of my stories. That gave Karen and me hope. But after seven months of working on the revised version of my book, and working as a basketball referee at night to make ends meet, it all ended. My computer destroyed every word I had written. In a panic, I stupidly loaded my backup disk onto the machine, thinking I could fix it. I couldn't. It destroyed that, too.

I became depressed. Karen finally gave up on me. I'd been telling her for a while that she deserved someone better than me, and I guess she finally took it to heart. She began going out with a customer at work, and then moved in with him.

The next ten days were among the most difficult I'd ever experienced. The world I had built for myself had come crashing down. The woman I loved had left me for a member of the Rahjneesh cult. My book was in terrible shape. I could hardly get through a day. Karen was my best friend and confidante, and she occupied my every thought from day to night. I hardly ate a thing. Karen refused to take my calls, but I finally persuaded a coworker to put her on the phone. I begged her to come back. She wouldn't. She sounded like a different person. I knew it was over.

I decided to leave the city. I couldn't bear the thought of living in the same city without her. I gave the apartment and everything in it to her and her new boyfriend for $1,000 and moved to Santa Cruz, a hundred miles south, in October 1984. A magazine located there called *Bay Sports* had offered me a job as editor. I called them up and accepted it.

To distract myself from the pain and depression, I stayed as busy as possible. I worked out with weights. I rode my bike constantly. And I put in long hours at the magazine. It was the first job I'd had with regular hours—and a steady paycheck—in a long time.

But a few short months later the magazine folded. That forced me back into sports officiating. I had to fight and scrap just to keep myself fed. And a volunteer job as the editor of the newsletter for the bike club in Santa Cruz consumed a lot of my time, too.

I lived in the bomb shelter under the pool hall for about a year. It was then that I met an attractive blonde named Leslie who introduced me to the teachings of Ramtha. Ramtha was a several-thousand-year-old entity who claimed to be a spirit god and talked through a woman named J.Z. Knight. Leslie gave Ramtha seminars and workshops and sold Ramtha videos and audio tapes.

I went to a seminar and borrowed some of Leslie's materials. I discovered a being who radiated great love, and who seemed to be goading me to really challenge life. He seemed to be telling me that every difficult moment I had experienced had been designed to make me stronger. And it made me start questioning the purpose of the rest of my life even more.

Then I got an idea.

I decided that the best way I could challenge these teachings, put them to the test, would be another bike ride across the country. Only this time I'd do it right. I'd ride the recumbent bicycle I'd picked up several years ago. I'd need a lot of new parts for it, but the reclined position I sat in was a lot easier on my body. And I'd tow a small trailer. I would also do the ride to benefit the National Head Injury Foundation; I'd become involved with them a few years before and been impressed with their dedication. Maybe I could drum up some interest and draw some attention to the Foundation while I was at it.

I had nothing to lose, and plenty to gain, this time.

"I don't know, Krieg. That sounds too weird for me. Everything you got is falling apart." Jeff Napier owned a bike shop, and I had dropped in to see what he thought about my new quest.

Coming from Jeff, "weird" really meant something. He was the one that label was usually meant for. He conducted his life, and his business, in a way that was totally out of the ordinary. Not only did Jeff spend hours throwing juggling pins with his friends in the parking lot in front of his store, but he did many of his errands on a 27-inch-wheel unicycle. To top it off, he lived in his Volkswagen bus.

"What's so weird about it? I thought that trailer you made for me could stand up to industrial use."

"It can, but I didn't make it to haul across the United States. I mean, look at your wheels. I scrapped 'em off an old three-speed we had out in back. That thing's so high off the ground, it'll be all over the place in your first head wind. It's just an errand trailer."

"That's why I want to have someone drive my Volkswagen bus for a support vehicle."

"You're dreaming, Krieg. You need a mechanic for that, too. It's kind of like your recumbent, it's falling apart." Jeff laughed at his joke.

Jeff was in his early thirties, with hair that receded in front and was long in the back and short on the sides. He looked like a cross between a rock-and-roll star and an Appalachian hillbilly. His hands always had a light film of grease on them from working on bikes.

"Maybe you're right. I've been thinking that I might be able to get a bike sponsorship to fill in for my bike."

"Dream on. You've got to be a racer for that." He paused. "Okay, let's suppose you do get a bike, which is ninety-nine percent unlikely because recumbent makers are far and few between and they're usually too poor to give a bike away— then how're you gonna feed yourself? And if one does give you a bike, they're not gonna want you to sleep in cardboard boxes or wear your umpire clothes, 'cause that's the only thing I see you wear that ain't rags."

I could feel myself getting angry. Jeff always meant well, but his blunt style sometimes hurt. I forced myself to keep calm. I would prove him wrong.

"Well... then I'll just build everything I need." I was reaching, but I was determined to come out of this conversation ahead.

"Get outta here, Krieg. Besides, why would people just give you things?" One of Jeff's friends walked into the store. "Hey, Dan, Martin thinks people are going to give him money to ride his bicycle across the U.S."

Dan looked at Jeff, then at me, then smiled. "To each his own," he said.

"Dan, wanna throw for a while?" Jeff was obviously more interested in juggling than discussing my trip.

"I was gonna ask you the same thing. Let's go."

I followed Jeff out to the parking lot, trying to answer his question. "They'll give me stuff because I'm gonna do the ride for the National Head Injury Foundation."

"Well, that's different, I support that." Jeff and his friend started tossing their juggling pins back and forth. "Martin, throw that pin to me when I say ready. We're gonna try for five at once."

Jeff had tried to get me to resurrect my book many times before. He thought it was a story which needed to be told, and he had encouraged me often.

Jeff's eyes followed the flight of the four juggling pins that he and his partner were now tossing back and forth to each other. A passing car honked its approval.

"Okay... ready." Jeff gave me my cue.

The speed of both the pins and the two jugglers increased as they labored to keep all five pins in the air.

"Want to go for six?" I offered.

Just as I said that, all five pins tumbled to the ground. They looked at me accusingly.

I grinned. "Gotta get going, you guys. I've got a trip to plan."

I returned to my basement apartment five miles out of town later that afternoon. In its present incarnation, the Casa de Montgomery served as a dormitory-like apartment complex for the outer fringes of the Santa Cruz population. Because I worked nights as an umpire and referee, I usually enjoyed the daytime quiet.

Since Jeff had outlined my needs for me, I went to work. He had pointed out that my recumbent bicycle and trailer both needed work. Knowing I probably couldn't count on my Volkswagen bus for sag support, I knew I would once again need a tent, a stove, and a sleeping bag. And Jeff was right about my bike clothes. I needed to improve my riding wardrobe if I was going after sponsors.

Over the next few days I examined the problems and their possible solutions. Then I outlined the possible options on the used computer I'd recently bought. After a few days, I started writing detailed proposals. I felt confident that my needs would be met in this way—somehow God would help me find what I needed.

Jeff was planning to attend a big bicycle trade show in the Los Angeles area in January 1986. Something told me I had to make it down there. A few days before Christmas I stopped into Jeff's shop.

"Jeff, what's up. Listen, can you get me into that bike show in Los Angeles?"

"What for? You don't have a bike shop,"

"There might be some people there that can help me with my ride. I've been in touch with the National Head Injury Foundation and they're all excited about it. All I need is some equipment."

"You still gonna take your recumbent? I told you, that thing's falling apart."

"That's what I was thinking. I might be able to get a component maker to sponsor me so I can get all the worn-out parts replaced. You never know."

"You don't need components. You need a whole new bike. Your seat is all busted. Look at this thing."

"I can get this reinforced."

"If you're towing the trailer I made for you, you're gonna be four hundred pounds right there." He sighed and shook his head. "I don't know."

"Aw, come on, Jeff. I can do it. I've done it once already and I'm gonna do it again, I need the challenge. I'll do it on a tricycle if I have to." I needed his support, and I made sure my tone carried that message.

Jeff looked at me for a few seconds.

"Well, what we gotta do is print you up some business cards."

As I walked into the Anaheim Convention Center with Jeff a few weeks later, the bright lights, flashy colors, and vast array of leading-edge cycling products momentarily overwhelmed me. Models walking the showroom floor in the latest bike wear competed for my consideration with big-screen film clips of mountain bike action. Every display seemed carefully designed to capture my attention, and the noise level was numbing. By the end of the morning all of this sensory overload blended into one cacophonous mess. I still had problems sorting out things like this.

I found what I was looking for sometime in the early afternoon. The recumbent bicycles in VIA Cycles' small booth looked out of place in this array of high-tech, speed-obsessed machinery.

I looked closely at the sleek, graceful lines of their premier model. A burly, forty-ish man of average height and with curly hair and a thick mustache came over and greeted me. He had muscular forearms and callused hands. His name was Mark Hajek, and he was the bike's designer.

"Ever ridden one before? You can take it out in the back lot if you want," he offered.

"I've been riding them for about five years, but I sure don't ride one anywhere near as beautiful as this."

"Go on then, take it for a spin."

"Who knows? If it rides as beautiful as it looks, maybe I can get it reviewed in the bike club newsletter I edit. I've also got a column in this regional magazine up in Santa Cruz. Maybe I can work it into that, too."

As I rode it in the parking lot out back, I knew I had found my very own two-wheeled nirvana. I knew, however, that I would have to do the best sales job of my life to get it.

"Mark," I said as I parked the bike, "I'm going to leave you with some documents that I've worked up. I'm looking for a recumbent bicycle sponsorship for my ride across the U.S. this summer, and I'm wondering if you might be interested."

"Is your number here?" He took the packet from me.

"Sure is. Basically what I've done is I've kind of outlined what I want to do, what I need to do it, and the schedules involved. I've included some samples of my writing and some news clips about my last ride. There are also some testimonials in there about my rehabilitation."

"Rehabilitation?"

"Yeah, I was in a coma for two months, I was paralyzed, I even had last rites said over me."

"No kidding?" I could see that I had aroused his curiosity. "I'll call you, okay? Excuse me, Martin, I've got to get back to my customers."

We shook hands and I walked off to see more of the show.

I left my proposal with those I thought could benefit from my ride. Bellwether, a bicycle clothing manufacturer, and Cascade Designs, the makers of an insulated ground pad, both told me they would help me if I located a bicycle sponsorship.

On the long drive home with Jeff, I sorted through the piles of literature I had accumulated. It was exciting to know that there were actually people in the bicycle industry who wanted to help me get my story out there.

I waited for a couple of days before I called Mark at VIA Cycles. I didn't want to sound too desperate and eager. We talked for a while about the show, then I said, "Well, did you get a chance to take a look at my proposal?"

"Pretty impressive. But who's going to be building this trailer that you've got sketched out here? I don't think anybody's going to buy sponsorships on it unless it's really a class act."

"First I gotta figure out what kind of recumbent I'm riding, so I can figure out which mounting system I'm going to use."

"I tell you what... I'll only let you ride one of my bikes if you let me also build the trailer. I don't want this thing looking like some ragtag bomb going down the road. You're only going to get top performance if the builder also provides you with a trailer that's engineered to his bike."

I was overwhelmed. Mark had just told me that he would not only supply me with the cornerstone of my dream, but he would also supply me with a trailer to tow behind it. I took a deep breath and tried to hide my excitement.

"But can you have all that built by April 5? That's when I'm leaving." I tried to make it sound like this was just an everyday business transaction.

There was a silence on the phone. Had I said the wrong thing and screwed it up? Then he replied. "No problem."

Since Mark based his operation out of Houston, Texas, we spent the next twenty-five minutes discussing all the details and logistics that would be involved in working together. By the time we said goodbye, I could hardly contain my joy.

I called Jeff at his bike shop.

"Hey, guess what? VIA's going to sponsor me."

"That's great. You still gonna put your advertising billboards on that trailer I built for you?"

"Get this—they're building me a new custom trailer. Same color as the bike."

I spent the rest of that day and most of the next calling people with the news. Then I began serious planning.

Since I only had three months to satisfy my long list of needs and tie up loose ends, I planned my every waking minute. Because of the cheaper phone rates, I got on the phone every morning at 5:30 and started prospecting for help on the East Coast. My dream began to come true bit by bit as I described my needs to those at the National Head Injury Foundation and bicycle component and accessory makers. Somehow I even felt directed to call a few head injury care providers.

Because nearly all of them wanted to see something in writing, I began crystallizing even more of my dream on my computer. Because they wanted to see specifics, I put together itineraries and a detailed listing of everything I'd need. I mapped out my route and flagged each state head injury association that I would be visiting.

My ride would consist of two parts. The shakedown part of my ride, when I would be acid testing my new bike and trailer, would take me across the western half of the U.S. as far as Houston and VIA Cycles. Once I reached Houston, the public relations part of my ride would begin. By trying to satisfy potential sponsors, I was able to plan my trip down to the most minute detail. My first TransAmerica trip would look Stone Age in comparison.

I even showed them how many and what size nicad batteries I would need to run my recorder and portable computer, and how I proposed to charge them. Since I had already taken one cross-country trip, I listed items such as squeeze tubes for peanut butter, a candle lantern, and a collapsible water bag—which convinced potential sponsors that I knew what I was talking about. I even detailed how many haircuts I would need, how much film I would use, and how often I would need to do laundry.

I remembered some of the difficult situations on my last ride, and resolved to toughen myself up for what lay ahead. I began to spend nights in my sleeping bag on the linoleum floor of my kitchen. I took cold showers. I ate camp-stove meals. I never turned the heater on. On my bike rides through the Santa Cruz mountains, I psyched myself up for the big desert I knew I would have to push myself through. I even filled my water bottles with hot water.

Before and after my rides, I spent a lot of time on the phone. I called magazine and newspaper editors and pitched my dream to them. I offered to write articles about my ensuing ride. On that short notice, my brother's national magazine, *Trucks*, agreed to publish one of my stories, and several regional publications ran articles on me, too.

I addressed several local service clubs and charitable organizations and circulated my prospectus in the local business community. Santa Cruz Cyclery, Chi Pants, Bay Photo Lab, Telephone Pioneers of America, Bicycle Inn, Family Cycling Center, and Pacific Pack and Pants boosted my confidence even higher when they donated products to my dream. They were joined by several national sponsors like Grainaissance, Vitasoy, Eden Foods, Caribou, Bellwether, Bolle, and Thermarest.

Then I got the phone call that took the ride to a whole new level.

"Martin? Hi, this is Jack Barrette of New Medico Head Injury Systems in Boston. The people at National tell me you're leaving pretty soon for a coast-to-coast bike ride. How can we help you?"

His strong, cultured voice intimidated me. I visualized a powerful executive dressed in a pin-striped suit, his hair graying at the temples. His office probably overlooked the Charles River.

"Well, I do still have a very long list of needs," I said trying to summon my best King's English.

"What I want to know is, how can we get our company name associated with your ride?"

"I can put one of your decals on my bike trailer," I rummaged through my desk for the list I had worked up of prices and positions. I can get you an eight-inch circle for $300, a six-inch rectangle for $200, or I can get you on the flag for $250. Oh no, wait... Vitasoy already bought that."

"So the flag is gone. How about your clothes? What have you got worked up there?"

"Well, Bellwether is providing me with bike shorts and tights and leg warmers, so it looks like I'm pretty good there."

"How about if we take care of your upper body? We can silk-screen our logo on your bike shirts."

"You're a genius. I never even thought about selling sponsorships there."

"What I'll do then is have my assistant call you back this afternoon. You two can figure out what you're going to need for all types of weather while you're on your ride, and then we'll figure out a price. Then, as soon as we get you out here to the East Coast, maybe we can get you to visit some of our facilities."

We chatted a while longer. I hung up the phone wanting to kiss the ground. It seemed that each new day of my quest brought a new surprise. I was just beginning to realize the possibilities of what my life could represent to others.

With just a month and a half to go, I gave notice on my little apartment and moved into an old friend's extra bedroom in town. I had met Lisa Lewis at a masters swim practice at Harvey West Park one day when I'd been considering swimming as a part of my training regimen. Lisa had once swum at the Olympic trials. She made my short stay at her place a warm experience. She tolerated with a smile my incessant visitors and phone calls, and she let me take over her garage and part of her house with possessions that I had not sold or sent off to storage.

April 5, 1986, was the big day. There was a combination going-away/send-off party at the Santa Cruz Wharf, given for me by several friends. They'd posted notices, contacted friends and family, and notified the local media. After everybody wished me luck, I pedaled away from the crowd of about fifty well-wishers on the pier. I felt I had just gone through a dress rehearsal for the events ahead, for I was scheduled to speak before several head-injury groups along my route and I hoped there would be more along the way. But I had grown fond of Santa Cruz in the year and change I had lived there, and I was sorry to leave. It was a tough ride away from the pier.

I pedaled south along the bay toward Monterey, then on down the coast through Los Angeles and inland to Fountain Valley, where I stayed with the Sandhorst family. Don and Jean Sandhorst headed up the Southern California Head Injury Foundation, and they had organized a reception for me. After a couple of days there I headed east through the Southern California desert. I packed many of the same items for this trip as for the last, with one major addition—my briefcase computer. I was now a writer, and I intended to make use of it extensively. I even had a special solar battery charger on the trailer.

I loved my new recumbent. It was much more comfortable to ride than my Eisentraut had been, and it worked more of my body, including my abdominals. It was even faster on flats, since it was lower to the ground and was less wind-resistant. It was also safer, and I had greater stopping power since my weight was over the back wheel. And I could see a lot more, since I didn't have to work at holding my head up. The trailer VIA Cycles had designed and built was state-of-the-art. It was streamlined to minimize wind drag and downplay cross winds. I must have been quite a sight to folks unfamiliar with reclining-position bicycles.

I took Interstate 10 east. My ride along the highway shoulder went smoothly until I reached Banning. The

scorching asphalt caused my front tire to blow up. I had
already discarded my backup tire because it wouldn't seat
properly, so I booted the gaping hole with part of my canvas
tool bag. As a result, I would have to bump up and down
the next three hundred miles, all the way to Phoenix, where
I could get help.

A few hours later, my trailer suddenly began to careen
back and forth across the roadway behind me. Afraid that I
would be jerked off the bike and into the path of the next
speeding vehicle, my heart almost popped out of my chest.
My body tensed. What was happening behind me? Finally,
I came to a halt.

I leaned my bike against a mileage marker and caught
my breath. I got off and tried to figure out what had just
happened. The bike looked fine. The trailer looked fine. The
road looked clear, and there wasn't a soul in sight. Stalled
once again in the sweltering heat, I finally discovered the
culprit. The spring Mark had installed to prevent just such
sideways movements had broken. I was even more relieved
when I remembered he had supplied me with a stronger
backup spring in case the lighter one failed. Anxious to get
moving again so that I could use the slight breeze that
pedaling created to keep cool, I replaced the faulty part as
fast as I could and began again.

Soon the sun and wind began to take their toll on my
face. My cracked and blistered lips were painful to the touch,
and it hurt to touch them with food. The salt from the
packaged nuts that I liked to eat out here and the citric juice
from the oranges I had bought felt like hot needles of pain.
It hurt to smile or even take sips from my water bottle.

Somehow I made it to Twenty-nine Palms on Highway
62, just north of the Joshua Tree National Monument. My
maps showed me that the next available water was 110
miles away, just over the Arizona border in Parker. After a
night in the outlying desert there, I pressed on.

The empty beverage containers that littered the shoulder
along that jarring hundred-mile stretch were irritating. As I
looked at the roadside garbage that had refreshed countless
earlier travelers, I resented anyone who was not drinking
hot water. Even the decals on my bike gave in to the piercing
heat. The little stickers slid out of position and nearly melted
right off the bike's frame tubing.

In the middle of nowhere, I began listening to the Ramtha

tapes that Leslie had loaned me. They comforted me and helped distract me from the brain-frying road ahead. The words rang true out here, and somehow the desert allowed me to understand the message of the tapes better than ever before. I felt that my ride was protected, and that I would be safe.

I made it to my water stop in Parker, and in the days that followed, I pushed through the barren lands of Arizona, New Mexico, and western Texas, staying on Interstate 10 most of the way. I camped most of the time, since there were few towns and cities, and the state head-injury groups were not very well organized. In Phoenix a head-injury family put me up, and the guys at Landis Cyclery took care of my recumbent's 16 x 1³/₈" front tire.

"I can't believe how lucky you are," said the mechanic there. "Those things have to be special ordered, and some guy ordered one and never picked it up."

"You guys got a pop-riveter here also?"

Several hours later I rolled out of their shop. They had stayed past closing time to pop-rivet my trailer mount back together, get my front tire replaced and properly seated, and even mount a generator lighting system so that I could attack more of the desert by night.

From Phoenix I detoured onto Highway 60 through Superior to Globe, then on 70 down to Lordsburg, New Mexico. I pulled into Lordsburg around seven in the evening in the middle of a raging windstorm and set up camp on the grounds of an elementary school.

I awoke the next morning to the voice of a railroad bum who had climbed out of one of a nearby boxcars.

"Where you goin' on that thing?" asked Charley.

I looked out my tent door and up at the middle-aged man. "I'm riding across the United States."

"Yeah? I did that last year on this ladies' three-speed I picked up at a garage sale. I think I paid five bucks for it," he said casually.

A likely story, I thought. "A three-speed, really? What route did you take?"

"Aw, hell, I rode mostly Ten to Florida. I really enjoyed it. People stopped me and gave me money. It sure beat hitchhiking or riding freight."

I looked at him more closely. He seemed reasonably fit and tan. Maybe, but... "How'd you carry your gear?"

"Just strapped it on. This bike shop in Santa Barbara gave me an old paperboy rack before I left. It worked great; I was able to get all sorts of stuff on there."

"How'd you ride Ten? I thought it was an interstate."

"Well, if there's no other road, they gotta let you ride 'em. They kicked me off in Louisiana for a while, though."

"Didn't those bumps on the shoulder drive you nuts?"

"They didn't bother me too much. I just took my time, maybe sixty miles a day."

"God, how did long you ride for? Didn't that seat bother you?"

"Well, after the coffee shop opened up, I'd drink three or four cups of coffee and ride all day on and off till the sun went down. I was in no hurry."

"Where'd you camp at night?"

"Like I said, I usually threw my bedroll down in the parking lot behind the coffee shop."

Inspired by Charley's story, I rode to Texas that day—198 miles, all on Interstate 10. Outracing rainstorms, I pushed my cycle computer past 52 miles an hour on one stretch, even passing a few eighteen-wheelers. At the end of the next day I camped in a campground just beyond the city of El Paso.

Fort Hancock, Sierra Blanca, Van Horn, Kent, Balmorhea, Fort Stockton, Ozona, Sonora... West Texas was hot and endless. It may feel and look like it's flat in a car, but I found that most of that part of the Lone Star State is long, grinding hills on a bike.

Just past Junction, I detoured onto Highway 290 through Fredericksburg and Johnson City into Austin, where I stayed for a couple of days. The Texas Hill Country surrounding Austin was surprisingly green, lush, and hilly, and I enjoyed the break from West Texas. I continued on 290 into Houston.

I pedaled into Houston three weeks after I'd left Santa Cruz. I was anxious to put into practice what I had learned from my tapes and thoughts about unconditionally loving and accepting myself. I'd finally realized that I had to be able to laugh at myself if I wanted to grow and expand. I was eager to see if I could remember to savor the miracle that life is—even when people placed their demands on me. Would I have the presence of mind to recall the wonder of an insect's wings, or the smell of a fresh-cut flower?

By the time I rolled up to the Easter Seals building, where

Jean De Wilde, the THIF program director, had scheduled my speech, I felt like I had just returned from a religious pilgrimage. Like Moses, I had descended from the mountain top with a message to deliver to my head-injured brothers and sisters.

Before my ride, I had no idea what I would say at the speeches I had scheduled. But I felt now that I could find the words that would truly help others. I could see that my car wreck and the long journey it had started me on had been an opportunity to discover some of the secrets of living—chief among them how to truly love and accept myself.

I remembered how, once I grew out of my coma, my ability to improve correlated directly with how I felt about myself. As my self-esteem increased through the support of friends and family, so did the speed of my recovery. I was ready to show others the importance of this discovery.

Head injury survivors, their families, and health practitioners in the field greeted me as I rolled up to the building's entrance. They cheered as I got off my bike. As I spoke with Jean, I could feel them studying me for any tell-tale signs of my head injury. Some children played on my bike.

The program director ushered me and my bicycle into a meeting room full of folding chairs. By the time everyone was seated, I counted nearly one hundred curious, expectant faces.

I could see that most of the people in the group were not head-injured. Almost immediately I started to have doubts. Did I really have anything of value to say to these people? Was I even qualified to stand before them? Would they try to question the methods and techniques that I was proposing for their head-injured patients or family members? I tried hide my nervousness. And the sight of the head-injured members of the audience reminded me who I was there for. I cleared my throat and began.

"Welcome, my fellow head-injured alumni. I want you to take a look around you and see all the people that we've brought closer to an appreciation for the simplest of life's very basics. Look at all the love that surrounds us." I leaned against a table as I continued, trying to hide my initial nervousness. "I know you want to hear about my bike ride, but I'm not going to talk much about that, I'm going to talk about you. I'm going to talk about why we're better people. You know that us survivors—no, let me change that name, us champions—have had a rare opportunity to see life from a completely different perspective. We've had all of our bodily functions shut down so we can learn what it is like to truly feel, to sense things at a different level than most people."

I could see by the looks on some of the faces before me that the last thought was too complicated, so I said it a different way. "We're all all-stars in this room, and we've been given an opportunity to operate at a higher frequency than most people. Our accidents gave us the tools to tune in a little bit better than most, so let's remember to think of ourselves as champions because we have that ability, and not as morons because most people can't sense who we are.

"I'm sure all of you want to know about my head injury," I continued. I took a few minutes to explain to them what I had gone through before sharing what had worked for me.

"The first thing you've got to do is love yourself unconditionally. Does anyone know what that means?" I watched a few of the parents nod their heads. "It means loving yourself when you're doing great as well as when you're blowing it. It means getting rid of the little guilts that all of us seem to be governed by. It means not being hard on yourself because you don't think you read enough or you haven't finished this book or that magazine. How many people in this room use the word, 'should'? Let me get a show of hands."

Practically everybody in the room raised their hand.

"Get rid of it. Don't use that word." I paused as a few people laughed. "You just do what you do and you don't what you don't, that's all. You're as perfect as any of God's creatures in things you don't do, as you are in things you do. And when you can learn to truly love yourself, then you can truly love everyone else for their mistakes and victories, too.

"How many people in here haven't forgiven themselves for their car wreck or whatever else got them here?"

A couple people raised their hands.

"Forgive yourself. Another part of loving yourself is letting yourself make mistakes. Have you ever seen a baby try to learn how to walk and every time he falls down he says, damn, and shoves his fist into the floor? No. They just get up and keep on trying. That's how we learn. Or have you ever seen a bird try to fly and just lay around on the ground as if to say, that's it, I'm not trying again? I don't think so. Why then are we better, just because we're adults? We're not. Forgive yourself for blowing it. Accept your mistakes. You might even do well to laugh at them.

"Laugh at yourself. I have found that so helpful for me. Let me get a feeling for how many head-injured family members there are in this room. Can I get a show of hands on that one?"

Twenty or thirty people raised their hands.

"Bless you. You know that you're a part of this journey as well, don't you? How many of you let your child or daughter or brother or sister or whatever think that the world has come to an end just because they're laid up? How many of you, when you go to see them in the hospital, change to a grave, serious person whenever you're around them? Stop! That's not in our best interest. Make it light for us. Bring laughter. Remind us that there is more to the world than hospital white.

"We should coach all of our visitors in the same way. Encourage them to come. We need them. The more the merrier. But have them bring fun. My hospital experience was a huge comedy extravaganza. I couldn't wait to get out and be part of that on the outside."

I watched several of the audience members nod their heads. "Another thing—we can't be playing any of this victim stuff. We're champions. My car wreck was the best thing that ever happened to me. And those head-injured people that I've come in contact with over the years that are superstarring at what they do all have the same attitude.

"And for those of you who are looking for the wonder drug or the magical mystery healer to rescue you from your woes, stop looking. It doesn't exist. Because it all begins and ends with you. You've got to do it. No one's going to do it for you. The strength of your conviction, the strength of your belief to get you beyond this stuff, is what's going to get you where you want to be. How many people in this room have ever wanted anything so bad that they would be willing to die for it?"

I stopped. People looked at each other. No one raised their hand.

"That's how bad you've got to want to beat this stuff. You've got to pretend that you will die if you can't do something that your therapist asks you to do, for example. The victories that you learn very early on in this way build the kind of character that you will need to overcome the rest of your challenges. Even today, I use the memory of my therapy successes when a hill gets too steep or head winds or rain reduce my pedal speed to a crawl.

"There's a bad word going around head injury circles these days, and I've heard people using it a lot around here. Deficits. Do you know how powerful words are? They are continuously shaping the world around us, and when you dwell on your deficits, or worse yet fail to acknowledge the other areas in which you are victorious, then you're doomed to live a life full of negatives. If you truly want to get better, you shouldn't talk deficit. Dwell on that shoe you tied today, or the button you buttoned. Make a fuss over your advances."

I could feel my face getting hot as I spoke. It made me mad to see anyone set limits for anyone else. Almost everyone that I could see in the audience before me seemed to understand what I was saying. I truly felt that there was a higher power using me to speak to these people.

"Make your therapy time the Super Bowl. Psyche yourself up for it. Build your day around it. Make each and every moment that you spend with your therapist an event which has no equal. If it's a difficult movement, like in physical therapy, take it home or back to your hospital room and dream about the result you want. Let your desired outcome monopolize your every waking moment. Smell your victory. Eat with it. Listen to the words of praise it will bring. Watch the happy looks on the faces around you. Go to bed with that vision on your mind. How bad do you want it? Ask yourself that question.

"How many of you favor one arm or hand over the other? I know a lot us have experienced atrophy of one form or the other. And if we're ever going to get those arms or legs or hands or feet to come back to normal, we can't be favoring them. I suggest that you put yourself in what I call a performance box.

"If you've got an itch on your left leg and your left arm doesn't work as good as your right, don't go into automatic and just scratch it with your right hand. Try to make a conscious effort of scratching that itch with your left arm."

I shuffled through my list of recommendations as I watched a couple of people taking notes.

"If it's hard to fit a key into a lock because one hand or the other trembles, try to force yourself to use that problem hand until in time it becomes easier and easier. And it will.

"Count change with your bad hand. This is a great way to work on your dexterity. Open your own door. Scratch your own itch. And always try to remember to do it with your weak side.

"Live in the now. Try not to think about the past. Don't ever try to go backwards and say, 'If only I'd have done this or done that, I wouldn't be in this mess.' You did what you did and you do what you do. The only time is right now. And be here now because there is no tomorrow. Because when tomorrow comes it's right now.

"Going back to the Super Bowl... that's about time, too. If what your therapist is asking you to do is too much for you and you think, 'Aw, I'll just do it next time,' then what do you think you'll say when the next time comes? 'I'll do it next time' becomes a pattern from which you can never escape. The only time is right now.

I had a captive audience, so I decided to take a chance and throw in a little about good nutrition. I discussed the dangers of simple sugars, pointing to a table in the back of the room loaded with jelly rolls and other junk food goodies. Then I paused, took a sip of water, and found the last thing I wanted to talk about in my notes.

"I want to wrap up with a discussion of goals. How many of you have them? Can I get a show of hands?"

Many in the group raised their hand.

"How about written-down goals?"

Only three people raised their hands.

"It's real important to write down your goals. It really helps to put your dreams and your hopes, because that's all that goals are, into concrete. Makes them more real and attainable.

"Your goals must be attainable, but just a little bit out of reach, and you must never compare yourself to others as you go about achieving them. One thing that I used to do, and I still do it today so I can keep myself on a positive note, is to write down every night those wins and gains that bring me closer to my goals. Get a family member to help you go over them. And if need be, have them write them down for you.

"Give yourself little rewards for your wins, because success is made up of all the little victories that lead up to it.

"I want to close by saying thanks for letting me speak to you today. Remember, if you shoot for the moon and hit a bird, it's better than shooting for the ground and hitting a rock. Dream big dreams. Reach for high heights. Go for it."

I wrapped up my presentation with a wish list. I had decided on my way to Houston that I would ask the Texas Head Injury Foundation for a few things I needed. I asked for a new tape recorder so that I would not have to stop and get off the bike to change sides. I asked for everything from a haircut to a pair of lightweight surgical pants. I told them that my stove had broken. I said that in a perfect world, I would also like a set of strapless pedals and shoes.

I could not believe my ears when one by one someone got up and offered to satisfy each and every one of my requests. Not only did the THIF save me money and the time and inconvenience of tracking down these items, but they even donated several hundred dollars more to my ride. This unexpected response to my talk overwhelmed me. They were telling me that my efforts mattered.

As I started to walk from the podium, my small audience got up and started clapping. I felt incredibly happy. I felt so much love for each and every one of them. Jean asked me if I could answer questions from the group, and for the next twenty-five minutes I talked about the specifics of my recovery.

Next on the agenda was Mark Hajek, the builder of my bike. He also gave me a hero's welcome. He replaced the bike he had shipped to me with a brand-new one. I stayed overnight at his house, his children made greeting cards for me, and his wife prepared delicious macrobiotic meals.

Mark even took time away from his busy bicycle business to take me down to Galveston, where I addressed a head-injury care facility called the Transitional Learning Center. I knew that my head-injured brethren were in good hands there; the TLC people were as excited to see me as their clients were.

After a few days of rest in Texas, I was ready for the second phase of my journey. I felt more confident than ever. I was riding the best touring machine in the world as an ambassador for the National Head Injury Foundation, and I was eager to do as much as I could for them.

Chapter 11

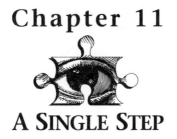

A SINGLE STEP

Seven years earlier, during my 1979 crossing, the focus of my ride had changed as I had gradually left the desolate states of the West and begun to travel through more densely populated areas. After Houston, the same thing happened on this ride. Added to that factor were several others: the new bike, the new pedals and cleats, and the moral support I'd received from my THIF presentation. The second half of my ride became the celebration I had always envisioned. And once I crossed over the Mississippi River, the media also took an interest in what I was doing.

I took Highway 59 north from Houston to Livingston, then turned east on Highway 190 to Jasper, Newton, and over the Louisiana border to Merryville and De Ridder. The beauty, water, and greenery of East Texas surprised me, and the luscious scenery continued into Louisiana. I cruised into Alexandria, then up Highways 28 and 84 into Jonesville and Vidalia and across the Mississippi River into Natchez. I traveled the Natchez Trace Parkway up along the Mississippi into Jackson. There I led several thousand bike riders through the rainy streets of the capital as a part of the Kodak bicentennial celebration. The Alabama Head Injury Foundation arranged TV talk show appearances and even more press for me on my way through their hilly state. Highway 20 was more or less a straight though extremely hilly shot over the Alabama border into Birmingham. There the Parker family generously accommodated me and took me around to the various head-injury rehabilitation centers. I met fellow survivors, their families, neuropsychologists, and physical and speech therapists.

Something I hadn't experienced before began happening. Drivers who had seen me on TV or in the newspapers began to stop me and ask for autographs as I headed north through Tennessee. Many even gave me money. The media was beginning to pay attention, and their coverage was paying off.

The riding itself, however, soon bored me, and for the first time during the ride, I began to question the value of my journey. Was I doing something that would benefit the thousands of misunderstood head-injured people throughout the country? Despite the media coverage, I wasn't sure I was making a difference. The answers I gave to the media in response to their questions began to sound trite and banal. I wondered how my story and my words could help other brain-injured people. What could I do out here on my bike? I tried to overcome the monotony of the ride by coming up with creative answers to already familiar questions—answers that would make a difference in the way our nation viewed the problem of head injury.

The attention intensified as I headed farther north through Alabama and into Tennessee. I pedaled into Knoxville, then north on Interstate 75 to Lexington and Cincinnati. The Kentucky Head Injury Foundation put me up in the first hotel of my ride and arranged for hospital visits and even more press.

By the time I reached Riverfront Stadium in Cincinnati, I felt like a celebrity who could do and say no wrong. As soon as I crossed over the Ohio River and headed into the stadium parking lot toward a band of waiting reporters, I already knew what to say.

"Martin, earlier you said that two million people a year suffer a head injury and that there's one every fifteen seconds. What does that mean?" One TV reporter asked as the others all pointed their microphones and cameras at me.

"Well, it means that our modern medical machines are not saving the whole person."

"And what do you mean by the whole person?" another reporter from a different group of cameras asked.

"How good a job are we doing at saving anybody when more than seventy-five percent of those suffering traumatic brain injury, who once led productive lives, can never return to the work force? When someone sustains a head injury, their life is changed forever. On the outside, they may look fine, but the scars, which most people don't see until they take a closer look, are what I'm talking about. Have you ever seen a grown man overwhelmed by a bus schedule or a grocery list? Most people don't have a clue about what it's like to lose everything. I mean *everything*. My world, for example, became an instant 'can't.' Things we learn as children, like tying shoes or drinking from a glass, suddenly become major undertakings. Once a head-injured person gets through the physical obstacles, a whole new set of hurdles begins to prevail. A lot of head-injured, even though they can look fine, end up in prisons or psychiatric institutions because they fail to communicate in an acceptable way." I felt like I was finally able to express myself the way I wanted to. At times I felt swept up in the momentum of my own words.

"What can we do?" one reporter asked.

"We can ask our insurance companies and our political leaders to recognize some of the new kinds of treatments that speak to this problem. Head injury isn't even classified as a debilitation in many states, so you can't even get disability insurance or any kind of money for things like cognitive therapy or vocational rehab."

"Can you give us some kind of feel for what kinds of things you went through along this line?"

"I can't tell you how dehumanizing it was for me to be in the middle of a sentence and have people walk away thinking I was on drugs or something. I also had a lot behavior problems. I laughed at the wrong times. I cried a lot. I interrupted conversations all the time. I was impetuous. I did and said things without ever thinking about the consequences. I couldn't hold onto a job because I was a behavior problem. But I will say one thing, us head-injured get better every day—we sure can't get any worse." That brought a laugh.

"You look and sound great to me. Sounds like it just took time for you. Won't most just get better over time?" Another member of the press asked.

"Every head injury is different. Every personality that it involves is different. I've been a fighter all my life. My whole life had been preparing me for a battle as grand as head injury. Even though I spent almost two months in a coma, the way in which it affected my operating center was different than the way it affects others. I know that I'm an exception to the rule."

They wanted to know what it was like to be in a coma; I told them. Then there was a question about my dying in the hospital.

"Well, I'll tell 'ya... I'm not afraid of it anymore. As the priest was saying last rites over me and everyone was looking sad, and my mom was crying and everything, I could feel myself saying, 'Aw, come on you guys, its not that big a deal.' I could almost feel myself asking them to join me. It was kind of a neat feeling. I had no worries, I was in a total place of surrender... I just did not care. I remember feeling kind of warm, and everything was real bright. And I guess it was at that point that I must have turned it all around, because I remember a voice asking me if I wanted to use my life to show people that we shouldn't take everything so seriously. And I said yes, and that was kind of when some of my numbness started going away. It seemed like the light began to lose some of its brightness. I began to feel irritable."

When I finished I wondered how much of what I had just said would make it to the nightly news. Was it a little too far out for my audience here? I had often spent several hours helping the TV news crews record a piece for the evening news only to find that they had used less than a minute of our work.

After the press conference was finished, the McNeil family, from the Ohio Head Injury Foundation, packed me and my bike into their van and took me to their home. There I met their head-injured son and rested up for my speech that evening.

After my warm reception in Cincinnati, I moved on to Columbus, where the ride changed once again. The very active Ohio Head Injury Foundation managed to get my story into the Associated Press and onto CNN. My story was now finding audiences throughout the nation.

I was in the OHIF office in Columbus when the phone rang for me.

"Hi, Martin. This is Peter Gilsey from New Medico. I'm glad I finally caught you."

"Caught me?"

"Yes, I've been trying to get a hold of you since you left Alabama. Of course the Tennessee head injury group doesn't seem very active, and you were almost in Ohio by the time you reached Lexington."

"Yeah, you're right, Tennessee was pretty dead. But I did meet a woman in Knoxville who helped me get in the newspaper there."

"Well, Martin, I've got good news for you. I've been hired to publicize your ride now that you're near our Pittsburgh facility."

It seemed that every time New Medico called, they were rewarding me with incredible news like this.

"Are you serious?" I felt an instant liking for this man. I sensed that he would work hard for me. There seemed to be a smile in his words.

"I sure am, Martin. But there is one catch. You've got to be willing to wait another few weeks before you head back home."

"Why's that?"

"Well, after you reach New York City for the Statue of Liberty Centennial celebration, we've got three facilities up in the Northeast that we'd like you to visit. If you can do it, then we've got to get them all set up. Then we'd like you to come up to see us in Lynn, just outside of Boston, and we're going to see if we can't arrange for you to meet Governor Dukakis at a State House press conference."

I was finally hitting the big time. Well, if they wanted me bad enough they'd have to take care of me. "If you guys want me to spend that much longer on the road, I'm not going to be scrapping for a roof over my head like I've been doing. I won't have any more state organizations expecting me."

"Can't you just camp?"

"The closer I get to the East Coast, the harder it is to find camping. There's just too many people and houses and buildings too close together."

There was a pause. "So what do you propose?"

"I'll finish the ride for you if you'll pay for me to stay in motels the rest of the way from New York."

"Hmm... I can't answer one way or the other on that, but let me check with Jack and call you tomorrow. Where are you going to be?"

"Somewhere between Columbus and Pittsburgh."

Peter laughed. "No wonder I had such a hard time getting a hold of you. Why don't I give you an 800 number and you call me at, say, two o'clock tomorrow. I'll have an answer by then. Does that work for you?"

Peter and I would get to know each other well over the next month as I called him regularly from roadside telephones along the way. We laughed as we compared his air-conditioned office to my outdoor surroundings. Our conversations always included a live update on such things as how many trucks were parked nearby, who was buying what, the numbers of other telephones in use around me, the outside noise level, or what the women within my sight looked like.

The first celebration he arranged for me was at their Cannonsburg facility just outside of Pittsburgh. I helped him set it up on the way in. I asked Peter if he could arrange a police escort. Somehow he pulled it all together in less than a week, and as a result established a template for the rest of my New Medico visits. After meeting the police car, I pedaled up the small hill to the Cannonsburg New Medico facility amid cheering and applause. As soon as I reached the wheelchair entourage, a brightly colored assortment of balloons floated up to the light blue sky. The fifty people who had assembled for the event all looked at me in awe. Several news reporters pressed in and began asking questions.

As we moved indoors to the cafeteria, which had been handsomely reappointed for me, I felt immensely proud. And I felt intensely grateful.

The Cannonsburg reception made the extra effort I had gone to seem worthwhile. After I gave my speech and visited patients, I stayed in a beautiful hotel near Pittsburgh over the weekend. New Medico shuttled me and my bike into the three-river city for interviews with the press, a photo session at a health fair, and a just-for-fun visit to an arts and crafts fair. Back at my hotel, everyone knew who I was. At the swimming pool, New Medico picked up the tab for all of my food and drink. They commissioned a machinist to make a new swing arm for my trailer. They even took me out for dinner and an evening of horse racing.

The rest of Pennsylvania was endless up-and-down riding. In its more densely populated areas, I competed for my share of the road with hostile, indifferent drivers. When I finally reached the New Jersey state line, I called my brother, Chris, who now lived in New York City.

Chris' life had changed a lot since our car wreck. Inspired by the advances I had made with my recovery, Chris had worked hard at making something of his own life. He had cofounded *Trucks* with a friend, and he was now an editor there. His risky journey east to make something of himself seemed incredibly adventurous to me. I wanted to impress him.

"Hey, Chris, this is Martin. Guess where I'm calling you from?"

Trucks had wanted to do an update on the article they had run before my ride, so I had called him once at the halfway point.

"I don't know... the last time I heard from you, you were in Texas. Let me guess—Kentucky."

"No way. Try New Jersey."

"New Jersey, are you serious? What part?"

"State line, somewhere east of Emmaus."

"I don't believe it! That's just a few hours away. Marty, I mean Martin, you're incredible. How you gonna get through the tunnels to get here?"

"Tunnels?"

"Yeah, where you at? How about if me and John come and get you? You're not that far."

"Under normal circumstances I'd say no. But I'm not done when I get to New York. I still have four more states to ride through for New Medico. They want me to tour their area for them. I could use a little rest, I guess."

A short while later I watched Chris as he and John, his partner in the magazine, pull into the parking lot. He looked pale as he climbed out of their company van. He seemed to be struggling with how to approach me. Did he think I'd come to haunt him, to dredge up memories of the car wreck that he'd tried so hard to forget?

We had grown apart through the years. Even though I'd forgiven Chris for his part in the accident, a small and irrational part of my mind still blamed him. And now I could feel part of me hoping he felt guilty.

He walked over, and we shook hands.

"You made it. You really are incredible."

"No big deal," I said. "I told you I would." Chris sensed that I wanted to keep him at a distance. I could see the disappointment in his eyes. We made small talk about the area, then Chris waved to my bike.

"Ready to go?"

"Yeah... let's go."

While Chris and John worked day and night readying their next issue for the printer, I regrouped and organized for the rest of my ride at Chris's studio apartment. Peter at New Medico told me that the press here was uninterested in my story. The Statue of Liberty celebration was the talk of the town. So I just blended in with the teeming millions. The day of the event, boats filled the harbor, and people and music filled the streets. I rode my bicycle from one street party to the next, dancing at several.

The next day I called Chris at work. I told him I was leaving.

"Sorry I couldn't spend any time with you, Marty, but John and I gotta put this thing to bed. We're almost done. You sure you can't stick around for another day or two? Then I could show you around."

"Chris, I only came here for the Statue of Liberty Centennial. I didn't expect you to entertain me. I've got to get rolling again for New Medico. It was kind of different racing around in Central Park, though."

"Well, take care, Mart... in," I could hear the smile in his voice. "There, I got it right. Call me if you need any help."

By the time I left New York City, I felt refreshed and alive again. I was glad to be traveling. I headed out onto Long Island, surprised at the beautiful, green country so close to the steel, asphalt, and concrete of the city. When I finally reached Port Jefferson, I was so impressed that I made a mental note of how pretty it was. I could live and write here, I thought.

The ferry across Long Island Sound brought me back to the mainland, at Bridgeport, Connecticut. I started my short trek north up the Post Road toward Southington, where I was to make my first New Medico facility visit. Along the way, on the streets of Stratford and Milford, people waved at me and my decal-laden trailer.

Dusk was nearing as I pulled up to the hotel address I had been given. "THE NATIONAL HEAD INJURY FOUNDATION WELCOMES MARTIN KRIEG" read the hotel marquee. That was a sign in more ways than one, for the attention I got during my visit lived up to that guest-of-honor billing. At facilities in Southington and Forestville, Connecticut, and Hyannis, Massachusetts, I talked to reporters and to patients and their families. I recommended building a head-injury hospital that would employ the latest research, equipment, and technology and be staffed by the best physicians, neurosurgeons, and therapists.

From Hyannis, I rode without the distraction of cars all the way to Provincetown at the tip of Cape Cod. The path I biked had been reclaimed from an old rail bed. It spread six or eight feet across, passing quiet lakes and picturesque cabin retreats.

I gave my imagination full rein here. What would I do when this final leg of my journey was complete? How could I use the energy of a story that had been witnessed by close to forty million people through the various media? Was helping to build a head-injury hospital really consistent with what I was all about? Was that the right way to channel my efforts, for the best return?

Then it hit me. Bike riding had been so beneficial for me in my rehabilitation. Not only was it good for my physical therapy, but my long rides had helped me sort out and process so much information that had overwhelmed me at first. How about a bike trail across the nation that head-injured people and bikers everywhere could use in their physical and mental therapy? On a larger scale, I knew that such a pathway would also improve the well-being of our nation in many ways.

The idea was so powerful that I had to stop my bike. I sat down and gazed over a small lake along the way. To reach such a goal, I knew I would have to acquire a lot of business skills and build an organization. And though I was sure that it was an idea whose time was coming, I knew it could take years before the need for such an important right of way would sink into the country's consciousness.

But the power and beauty of the vision were overwhelming and extremely exciting. Having crossed the country twice on a bike, I knew better than anyone how badly a biking path was needed. And finally, it would give me another challenge.

For now, however, I had to finish my ride. I spent the night in an inn at Provincetown. The next morning I took the ferry over to Boston. I was filled with doubts. Would New Medico's Jack Barrette even approve of what Peter and I had accomplished over the last month? And how about Governor Dukakis? Would he really show up?

After the boat docked, I pedaled the short distance to the capitol building. Along the way, cars honked and people cheered. A man in a taxi asked for my autograph. He said he had seen me on the news a few nights before.

As I rolled up the hill to the small crowd assembled in front of the State House, I recognized Peter right away by his big smile. He looked out of place in his suit; his shaggy blond hair and fit physique made him look as if he would be more at home on a surfboard.

"I'll bet you're Peter," I said as I reached my hand out to shake his.

His smile grew larger. "How did you know?"

"Oh, I could sense it. You looked proud of what you had done."

"No, you did it, Martin. But I will tell you, we had some moments back there. Getting you accommodated was a logistical nightmare, trying to use a road map and a pay phone sometimes."

We both laughed. "Is the governor still going to be here?" I asked.

"He sure is. But before we do anything, let's let you answer some of these reporters' questions, okay? Oh, and Martin, do you recognize this guy?" Peter grabbed the arm of a tall, square-shouldered man next to him.

"I don't think so," I said as the small band of reporters pressed even closer.

"This is Jack Barrette."

I took a good look at him. He seemed much warmer and younger than the man I had pictured during our conversations months earlier.

"Thanks for making this ride possible, Jack. I'm truly grateful."

"No, thank *you*. You and Peter did a really superb job."

I turned my attention to the press and answered their questions. Then Governor Dukakis and his wife, Kitty, came out to the front steps and posed with me and Marilyn Spivack, the founder of the National Head Injury Foundation. Cameras flashed and TV equipment moved into position as the governor shook my hand and introduced me to his wife.

As I looked into the cameras, I thought about all the people whose lives I had touched. I thought about Rich Milan and how he had refused to let me just laze around, and Don Chu and his staff. My uncle Jam had helped me regain my confidence and sharpen my mind, and Angelo had done the same for my body.

I felt blessed to have been loved and cared for by Janice and then Karen. My brother Chris had helped me to see how far I could push myself in the hospital, and I knew that he had always tried to help me even when I was pushing him away. My sisters Kathy, Nancy, and Karen had never let me forget the love that they had for me. And my mother had always been there for me, no matter what my problem.

I knew now that the difficult situations and people I had encountered had only strengthened me. I knew without Dad's stern approach I would have given up a lot easier. Bob and Jeff were only verbalizing what I knew inside to be true.

These people and the many others who had touched my life would always be with me.

I resolved that, no matter how many years it took, building a coast-to-coast bicycle greenway would be my next goal. It would be a proper way to honor all of those people. And finally, I actually felt grateful for my car wreck. Without it, I would never have grown as much as I had, never have understood myself as well and come to terms with that understanding. I had finally come to love and accept myself, and I had come a long way from the skinny, insecure kid I'd been. I felt like my recovery was complete. I was happy with who I was.

I knew if I could do what I'd done, beat my head injury with the help of others, I could rally people around something of importance to all of the planet, and its children and its children's children.

The words of the sixth-century Chinese philosopher Lao-tzu went through my mind: "The longest journey begins with but a single step."

I knew I had already begun.

Afterword

GREENWAY 2000—
A VISION FOR AMERICA

Since 1987, Martin Krieg has dedicated himself to his vision of a coast-to-coast, multi-use transportation and recreational bicycle trail—the National Bicycle Greenway. The primary purpose of the Greenway is to provide a safe, clean, aesthetic, and enjoyable place for people of all ages to bike year-round. This uninterrupted right-of-way will make the joy of bicycling more available for many Americans. In addition, it will reconnect us with nature and our neighbors, promote better health, and address many of our pressing environmental concerns.

The Greenway will utilize a network of abandoned rail lines and highways as well as active utility and aqueduct rights-of-way. It will ultimately be fed by other bicycle highways that stretch up and down both seaboards and crisscross America from east to west and north to south.

Design and construction firms that specialize in bicycle trails will emerge as the Greenway program unfolds. Since the Greenway will be tastefully designed in a linear, park-like setting, service crews will maintain the landscaping, signage, rest areas, and information kiosks that will border this important arterial.

Restaurants, lodging, and other support services will spring up along the Greenway, creating new jobs, and the structures that support these services will be designed to enhance the natural character of the Greenway. Young people can find summer work transporting elderly and disabled people on bike taxis. A bike shuttle service will be available for transporting items that are hard to carry on a bicycle.

The Greenway will stimulate a whole new market for tourism domestically and from abroad. Periodic rest stops will give Americans more opportunity to meet each other and people from around the world.

This linear parkway will be used for commuting and recreation during the week, and on weekends, especially in urban areas, it will see additional use by roller skaters, hikers, joggers, and the physically challenged.

This motor-vehicle-free corridor will link our urban areas with our wilderness and other open-space lands, and it will be designed so that wildlife will be able to safely cross it. On the stretches between urban areas, markers along the Greenway will explain the history and geography of the various regions.

By underscoring the joy of riding a bike, and showcasing pedal power's ability to enhance health, save our natural resources, and reconnect us with nature, the Greenway will attract great numbers of people to bicycling in many different parts of America. In time, a network of bicycle greenways will help solve many of our traffic and air pollution problems as well.

In order to collect resources and energy for this vision, Martin founded a company in Santa Cruz, California, called Cycle America. Since 1987 he has been able to contract with some of the best graphic talent on the West Coast to publish regional bicycling guides in four different areas of California. Besides promoting the Greenway, these attractive, pocket-sized books use fold-out maps and up-to-date information to show cyclists where to ride, eat, sleep, shop, and play in each of the areas they serve.

With the recent incorporation of the nonprofit National Bicycle Greenway (NBG), his publishing company will expand as it becomes a part of the much larger NBG organization. Besides taking the directories to a national level, the NBG will also educate the public regarding a healthful, environmentally sound lifestyle and gather and coordinate the resources needed to create and maintain the Greenway.

Those interested in helping Martin actualize his dream can make tax-deductible donations to: The National Bicycle Greenway, 147 River Street South, Suite 222, Santa Cruz, CA 95060. If you would like more information, call (408) 426-7702 or (408) 425-8533 (fax).

To further promote the National Bicycle Greenway,
Martin would like to take hundreds of cyclists with him
on another TransAmerica bike ride during the summer of 1995.
If you would like to join with this coast-to-coast celebration,
please inquire at the National Bicycle Greenway address listed above.

Suggested Affirmations

Because words have such a powerful impact on our lives, I use affirmations to help me move through many of life's challenges. I print them on little slips of paper and put them in places where I will see them over and over again, such as on my refrigerator door, light switches, bathroom mirror—even on the handlebars of my bicycle. You can make them pretty, if you like, with calligraphy or different-colored inks, or you can find someone with a computer who can output them from a desktop publishing program. As your life unfolds, different challenges will require different such reminders, so as you gain some measure of mastery, you will want to design your own. Just remember to make them positive, first or second person, and as concise as possible.

From the list below, determine which *one* area you most want to concentrate on and place the associated affirmation everywhere you can. I have set them up in the sequence that worked for me. If after a few days, weeks, or months, you feel you have internalized the needed words, replace them with words pertaining to the next area you want to master.

To be able to love and accept yourself...
　　I love and accept myself just as I am.

To have that love reflected back to you and to quit blaming yourself or others...
　　I bombard with love.

To realize that no wonder drug, therapist, or medical miracle is going to get you better...
　　I am created in the image of God; I can do anything.

To make the most out of therapy...
　　There is no tomorrow; the only time is now.

To put forth your best effort in any endeavor...
　　Push yourself.

To cope with the changed person you have become...
　　Be yourself.

To be willing to attempt that which you think could be good for you...
>There is no "try," there is only "do" and "not do";
>>and/or
>
>Do what you're afraid of and the fear will be replaced.

To accept the childlike mistakes you are bound to make...
>Laugh at yourself.

To keep pushing through the pain mistakes cause you...
>Love your mistakes; they bring you closer to the desired result.

To be an achiever...
>Do it now.

To make life a truly grand adventure...
>I look for joy; I expect the best.

To have fun...
>I now deserve fun;
>>and/or
>
>LAUGH!

To understand how you create the circumstances that come your way...
>What is my belief system about it?

To learn what you want to focus your energy on...
>Get clear.

To remind yourself that you're special...
>I am blessed.

To remind yourself that you have no limits...
>I am a spiritual being having a human experience.

A PROPER MENTAL DIET

If you take a glass of dirty water and keep filling it with clean water, the water ultimately becomes clean. Somewhere within, I knew the mind of man operated in the same way. Since I had been given a chance to start over, I substituted the following books for the newspapers I used to read and the television I used to watch:

I found that *PsychoCybernetics* by Maxwell Maltz helped me to improve the way I thought about the more limited person I thought I had become, while Wayne Dyer in *Your Erroneous Zones* showed me that I was the only one in charge of my life or my feelings. Dale Carnegie, in his classic, *How to Win Friends and Influence People,* gave me some excellent ideas on how I could use my new personality to get along with people.

In redefining myself as a complete person and not as a cripple, *Think and Grow Rich* by Napolean Hill and *Success Through a Positive Mental Attitude* by W. Clement Stone challenged me to raise what I expected from life. *The Magic of Thinking Big* by David M. Schwartz aggrandized these visions even more.

Personal Power Through Awareness by Sanaya Roman showed me how to best work with my own energy and that of others, while one of her other books, *Spiritual Growth,* helped me to function more as my Higher Self. Wayne Dyer, with *You'll See It When You Believe It,* reinforced the fact that we are really spiritual beings first and physical beings second. His most recent book, *Real Magic,* then proves that we have no limits when we come from these higher realms.

Denis Waitley's tape series, *The Psychology of Winning,* impregnated my consciousness with the kind of thoughts I would need to become a winner in the game of life. As Ramtha, channeled by J.Z. Knight, downsized her operation after my 1986 ride, I discovered Sanaya Roman's company, *Luminessence,* in Oakland, California. Besides the books I've already mentioned, Sanaya and Duane Packer have used their guides to channel excellent tapes on everything from abundance to relationships to starting your own business.

The X-factor in my rehabilitation was nutrition. Instead

of fine-tuning my motor skills after my 1979 ride, I found myself fighting colds, flu, and sore throats until I changed the way I nourished myself. Since 1980, I have also watched my mental acuity grow by following a macrobiotic diet and I think of the discipline needed to maintain it as a form of health insurance. Any of Michio Kushi's many books, including *The Standard Macrobiotic Diet* and *The Macrobiotic Way*, as well as *Introduction to Macrobiotics* by Carol Heidenry do a good job of introducing one to this new way of eating and living.

Because experience has taught me that we create our lives with the thoughts we think, I resort religiously to Louise Hay's little book, *Heal Your Body*, in order to identify those thought forms that introduced even the slightest ache, bump, or irritation to my life.

A NOTE ON THE NATIONAL HEAD INJURY FOUNDATION

Serious head injuries usually result in prolonged loss of consciousness or coma. While it may be brief, lasting only a few minutes, unconsciousness may extend to days or weeks. As time in coma lengthens, emergence to a fully alert state is less likely and the victim will suffer intellectual impairment, speech problems, and physical disorders. The individual and his family face a period of rehabilitation that can last for years.

It is estimated that 100,000 persons die annually from head injuries in the United States and that over 700,000 have injuries severe enough to require hospitalization. Of this group, between 50,000 and 90,000 people a year are left with intellectual or behavioral deficiencies that prevent them from returning to normal life. Two-thirds of these people are below the age of 30.

The National Head Injury Foundation (NHIF) is a national advocacy group working to prevent head injuries and to provide support to head-injured survivors and their families. The group distributes literature, advocates legislation, raises money for research, and assists in the establishment of rehabilitation programs.

THE NATIONAL HEAD INJURY FOUNDATION MISSION STATEMENT

The mission of the National Head Injury Foundation is to ADVOCATE for and with people who survive traumatic brain injury, to secure and develop community based SERVICES for survivors of traumatic brain injury and their families, to support RESEARCH leading to better outcomes that enhance the life of people who sustain a brain injury, and to promote PREVENTION of brain injury through public awareness, education, and legislation.

The National Head Injury Foundation is a not-for-profit organization, located at 1776 Massachusetts Avenue, N.W., Suite 100, Washington, D.C. 20036. Phone (202) 296-6443, Fax (202) 296-8850, Family Help Line 1-800-444-NHIF.

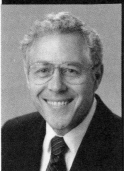
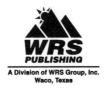